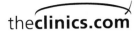

RHEUMATIC DISEASE CLINICS OF NORTH AMERICA

Antiphospholipid (Hughes) Syndrome

GUEST EDITOR
Munther A. Khamashta, MD, FRCP, PhD

August 2006 • Volume 32 • Number 3

SAUNDERS

An Imprint of Elsevier, Inc.
PHILADELPHIA   LONDON   TORONTO   MONTREAL   SYDNEY   TOKYO

W.B. SAUNDERS COMPANY
A Division of Elsevier Inc.

1600 John F. Kennedy Boulevard • Suite 1800 • Philadelphia, Pennsylvania 19103-2899

http://www.theclinics.com

RHEUMATIC DISEASE CLINICS OF NORTH AMERICA August 2006 Editor: Rachel Glover	Volume 32, Number 3 ISSN 0889-857X ISBN 1-4160-3903-1

The ideas and opinions expressed in *Rheumatic Disease Clinics of North America* do not necessarily reflect those of the Publisher. The Publisher does not assume any responsibility for any injury and/or damage to persons or property arising out of or related to any use of the material contained in this periodical. The reader is advised to check the appropriate medical literature and the product information currently provided by the manufacturer of each drug to be administered to verify the dosage, the method and duration of administration, or contraindications. It is the responsibility of the treating physician or other health care professional, relying on independent experience and knowledge of the patient, to determine drug dosages and the best treatment of the patient. Mention of any product in this issue should not be construed as endorsement by the contributors, editors, or the Publisher of the product or manufacturers' claims.

Rheumatic Disease Clinics of North America (ISSN 0889-857X) is published quarterly by Elsevier Inc., 360 Park Avenue South, New York, NY 10010-1710. Months of issue are February, May, August, and November. Business and editorial offices: 1600 John F. Kennedy Boulevard, Suite 1800, Philadelphia, PA 19103-2899. Customer Service offices: 6277 Sea Harbor Drive, Orlando, FL 32887-4800. Periodicals postage paid at New York, NY and additional mailing offices. Subscription prices are USD 190 per year for US individuals, USD 305 per year for US institutions, USD 95 per year for US students and residents, USD 225 per year for Canadian individuals, USD 370 per year for Canadian institutions, USD 250 per year for international individuals, USD 370 per year for international institutions and USD 125 per year for Canadian and foreign students/residents. To receive student/resident rate, orders must be accompanied by name of affiliated institution, date of term, and the *signature* of program/residency coordinator on institution letterhead. Orders will be billed at individual rate until proof of status received. Foreign air speed delivery is included in all *Clinics* subscription prices. All prices are subject to change without notice. POSTMASTER: Send address changes to *Rheumatic Disease Clinics of North America*, Elsevier Periodicals Customer Service, 6277 Sea Harbor Drive, Orlando, FL 32887-4800. **Customer Service: 1-800-654-2452 (USA). From outside of the USA, call (+1) 407-345-4000. E-mail: hhspcs@harcourt.com.**

Reprints. For copies of 100 or more of articles in this publication, please contact the Commercial Reprints Department, Elsevier Inc., 360 Park Avenue South, New York, 10010-1710; Tel.: (+1) 212-633-3813, Fax: (+1) 212-462-1935, and E-mail: reprints@elsevier.com.

Rheumatic Disease Clinics of North America is covered in *Index Medicus, Current Contents/Clinical Medicine, Science Citation Index, ISI/BIOMED,* and *EMBASE/Excerpta Medica.*

Printed in the United States of America.

GUEST EDITOR

MUNTHER A. KHAMASHTA, MD, FRCP, PhD, Director, Lupus Research Unit, The Rayne Institute, King's College London School of Medicine, St. Thomas' Hospital, London, United Kingdom

CONTRIBUTORS

MARY-CARMEN AMIGO, MD, FACP, Associate Professor of Rheumatology, Universidad Nacional Autónoma de México Department of Rheumatology, Instituto Nacional de Cardiología Ignacio Chávez, Mexico City, Mexico.

RONALD A. ASHERSON, MD, FRCP, FACP, Division of Immunology, School of Pathology, University of the Witwatersrand, Johannesburg, South Africa

MARIA LAURA BERTOLACCINI, MD, PhD, Louise Gergel Postdoctoral Research Associate, Lupus Research Unit, The Rayne Institute, King's College London School of Medicine at Guy's, King's and St. Thomas' Hospitals, St. Thomas' Hospital, London, United Kingdom

RICARD CERVERA, MD, PhD, FRCP, Department of Autoimmune Diseases, Hospital Clínic, Barcelona, Catalonia, Spain

ROLANDO CIMAZ, MD, Département de Pédiatrie, Hopital Edouard Herriot, and Université Claude Bernard- Lyon 1, Lyon, France

DAVID D'CRUZ, MD, FRCP, Consultant Rheumatologist and Honorary Senior Lecturer, Louise Coote Lupus Unit, St. Thomas' Hospital, London, United Kingdom

MARIA JOSE CUADRADO, MD, PhD, Consultant Rheumatologist, Louise Coote Lupus Unit, St. Thomas' Hospital, London, United Kingdom

ELODIE DESCLOUX, Service de médecine interne-pathologie vasculaire, Centre Hospitalier Lyon Sud, France

DORUK ERKAN, MD, Assistant Attending Physician, Hospital for Special Surgery; Assistant Professor of Medicine, Weill Medical College of Cornell University, New York, New York

JOSEP FONT, MD, PhD, FRCP, Department of Autoimmune Diseases, Hospital Clínic, Barcelona, Catalonia, Spain

GRAHAM R.V. HUGHES, MD, FRCP, Lupus Research Unit, The Rayne Institute, King's College London School of Medicine at Guy's, King's and St. Thomas' Hospitals, St. Thomas' Hospital, London, United Kingdom

KAZUKO KOBAYASHI, PhD, Department of Cell Chemistry, Okayama University Graduate School of Medicine, Dentistry, and Pharmaceutical Sciences, Okayama, Japan

MICHAEL D. LOCKSHIN, MD, Professor of Medicine and Obstetrics-Gynecology, Hospital for Special Surgery, Weill Medical College of Cornell University, New York, New York

LUIS R. LOPEZ, MD, Corgenix, Inc., Westminster, Colorado

EIJI MATSUURA, PhD, Associate Professor, Department of Cell Chemistry, Okayama University Graduate School of Medicine, Dentistry, and Pharmaceutical Sciences, Okayama, Japan

HARALAMPOS M. MOUTSOPOULOS, MD, FACP, FRCP, Professor of Internal Medicine and Head of the Department of Pathophysiology, Medical School, National University of Athens, Greece

MICHELLE PETRI, MD, MPH, Professor of Medicine, Department of Medicine, Division of Rheumatology, Johns Hopkins University School of Medicine, Baltimore, Maryland

UMAIR QAZI, MD, MPH, Kirkland Scholar, Department of Medicine, Division of Rheumatology, Johns Hopkins University School of Medicine, Baltimore, Maryland

GIOVANNI SANNA, MD, FRCP, PhD, Consultant Rheumatologist, Department of Rheumatology, Homerton University Hospital, London, United Kingdom

MASAKO TABUCHI, MD, Department of Cell Chemistry, Okayama University Graduate School of Medicine, Dentistry, and Pharmaceutical Sciences, Okayama, Japan

MARIA G. TEKTONIDOU, MD, PhD, Consultant Rheumatologist, Department of Pathophysiology, Medical School, National University of Athens, Greece

FELICIA TENEDIOS, MD, Rheumatology Fellow, Hospital for Special Surgery, Department of Rheumatology, Weill Medical College of Cornell University, New York, New York

CONTENTS

The antiphospholipid syndrome (APS) is a systemic autoimmune disease clinically characterized by recurrent arterial or venous thrombosis or pregnancy complications including recurrent early miscarriages or fetal losses. The presence of antiphospholipid antibodies (aPL) is mandatory to make the laboratory diagnosis of APS. In clinical practice, the gold standard tests are those that detect anticardiolipin antibodies (aCL) by ELISA or the lupus anticoagulant (LA) by coagulation tests. Anti-β2GPI testing is also a helpful diagnostic tool for the APS, particularly when aCL and LA are negative and APS is strongly suspected. The clinical utility of other aPL specificities has still to be established.

In the early 1980s, Graham Hughes and his team published a number of studies that showed an association of antiphospholipid antibodies (aPL) with a wide range of neurologic features including stroke and transient ischemic attacks, and a variety of other neurologic syndromes. The antiphospholipid (Hughes) syndrome (APS) is today recognized as a major cause of neurologic disease. However, precise mechanisms of cerebral involvement in APS are still ill defined. aPL play an important role in the activation of endothelial cells in the cerebral vessels causing thrombosis and ischemic events. Alteration of the circulation of small vessels of the brain is likely to be responsible for some of these neurologic features, including seizures and cognitive dysfunction. Animal models are providing insight in a possible role of these antibodies in the production of direct neurologic tissue damage through immune-mediated mechanisms. In this overview of the cerebral manifestations of APS we will focus on the most relevant aspects for the clinician.

The antiphospholipid syndrome (APS) is characterized by the presence of circulating antiphospholipid antibodies (most commonly detected by a lupus anticoagulant test, anticardiolipin antibody ELISA, and anti-β2-glycoprotein-I antibody ELISA), vascular thrombosis, and/or pregnancy loss. Antiphospholipid syndrome is a systemic autoimmune disease with diverse clinical manifestations involving different organ systems. The cardiac system is one of the major target organs in APS.

The kidney is a major target organ in patients with the antiphospholipid syndrome (APS). The renal manifestations may result from thrombosis occurring at any location within the renal vasculature including glomeruli, arterioles, and parenchymatous arteries. It is unclear whether, in addition to thrombosis, other mechanisms could also contribute to the pathogenesis of the APS nephropathy. The characteristic APS vascular nephropathy features thrombotic microangiopathy, fibrous intimal hyperplasia affecting the interlobular arteries and their branches, and focal cortical atrophy. Systemic hypertension is a key clinical finding. Further studies are needed to understand the basic mechanisms of the renal involvement in APS and to define a rationale treatment.

Osteoarticular manifestations have been poorly recognized in antiphospholipid syndrome (APS). Arthralgias represent the most commonly described musculoskeletal manifestations of primary or secondary APS, while arthritis has been mainly reported in systemic lupus erythematosus (SLE)-related APS patients. Osteonecrosis has been described in association with antiphospholipid antibodies in patients with SLE or APS, as well as in several patients with nonautoimmune disorders.

compensate for excessive maternal bleeding during delivery. In addition, venous stasis due to venous dilation and compression of the uterus occurs, leading also to a higher risk of thrombosis. The goal of treatment of APS in pregnancy is to protect the mother from thrombosis and to reduce the risk of fetal loss.

Index

FORTHCOMING ISSUES

RECENT ISSUES

THE CLINICS ARE NOW AVAILABLE ONLINE!

Access your subscription at:
http://www.theclinics.com

ELSEVIER
SAUNDERS

Rheum Dis Clin N Am
32 (2006) xi–xii

RHEUMATIC
DISEASE CLINICS
OF NORTH AMERICA

Preface

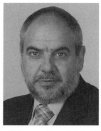

Munther A. Khamashta, MD, FRCP, PhD
Guest Editor

The antiphospholipid syndrome (APS), or "Hughes Syndrome," describes patients with a hypercoagulable disorder resulting in increased fetal loss and recurrent arterial or venous thromboses, often associated with thrombocytopenia and livedo reticularis, in whom antiphospholipid antibodies can be demonstrated. Correct identification of patients with this syndrome is important because prophylactic anticoagulant therapy can prevent thrombosis from recurring and treatment of affected women during pregnancy can improve fetal and maternal outcome.

It has been five years since the *Rheumatic Disease Clinics of North America* devoted an issue to this topic, and much new knowledge has been accumulated. New advances in clinical presentation and antiphospholipid testing, along with therapeutic approaches to patients with APS, including the catastrophic subset, are reviewed in this issue.

0889-857X/06/$ - see front matter © 2006 Elsevier Inc. All rights reserved.
doi:10.1016/j.rdc.2006.07.001   *rheumatic.theclinics.com*

Dedication

This issue is dedicated to Dr. Josep Font, a close friend and major contributor to the knowledge in this field.

Munther A. Khamashta, MD, FRCP, PhD
Lupus Research Unit
The Rayne Institute
King's College London School of Medicine
St Thomas' Hospital
London SE1 7EH, UK

E-mail address: munther.khamashta@kcl.ac.uk

ELSEVIER
SAUNDERS

Rheum Dis Clin N Am
32 (2006) 455–463

RHEUMATIC
DISEASE CLINICS
OF NORTH AMERICA

Antiphospholipid Antibody Testing: Which Are Most Useful for Diagnosis?

Maria Laura Bertolaccini, MD, PhD*,
Graham R.V. Hughes, MD, FRCP

*Lupus Research Unit, The Rayne Institute, King's College London School
of Medicine at Guy's, King's and St. Thomas' Hospitals, St. Thomas' Hospital,
London, United Kingdom*

The antiphospholipid syndrome (APS) is a systemic autoimmune disease clinically characterized by recurrent arterial or venous thrombosis or pregnancy complications including recurrent early miscarriages or fetal losses. The presence of antiphospholipid antibodies (aPL) is mandatory to make the laboratory diagnosis of APS. In clinical practice, the "gold standard" tests are those that detect anticardiolipin antibodies (aCL) by ELISA or the lupus anticoagulant (LA) by coagulation tests. Although other specificities for aPL have been described, their clinical utility has still to be established.

History of antiphospholipid antibodies

Wasserman [1] was the first to describe aPL, a complement-fixing antibody that reacted with extracts from bovine hearts, while carrying out his research into the development of the serologic test for syphilis. But only in 1941 was the relevant antigen identified as cardiolipin [2], becoming the basis for the Venereal Disease Research Laboratory (VDRL) test for syphilis. Blood screening for this disease led to the observation that many patients with systemic lupus erythematosus (SLE) had a positive VDRL test, without any other clinical or serologic evidence of syphilis [3].

The knowledge of the "lupus anticoagulant phenomenon" goes back to the 1950s when Conley and Hartmann [4] reported a prolongation of the prothrombin time in patients with SLE. In 1954, this "circulating

Maria Laura Bertolaccini is a Postdoctoral Research Associate funded by the Louise Gergel Fellowship.
* Corresponding author.
E-mail address: maria.bertolaccini@kcl.ac.uk (M.L. Bertolaccini).

anticoagulant" was associated with recurrent abortions [5], followed in 1957, by a report on its association with the biologically false-positive test for syphilis [6]. In 1963, the "circulating anticoagulant" was associated with thrombotic manifestations in SLE [7], but it was not until 1972, that Feinstein and Rapaport [8] introduced the term "lupus anticoagulant" and described it as an inhibitor directed against coagulation cascade phospholipids, particularly at the prothrombin conversion to thrombin step.

In 1983, Hughes [9] described in full clinical detail the APS (which he originally entitled "anticardiolipin syndrome"). His clinical observations included the tendency to both arterial and venous thrombosis, the "primary" syndrome in the absence of SLE, the livedo, thrombocytopenia, recurrent pregnancy loss, and prominent neurologic involvement. This group set up a sensitive solid phase immunoassay for the detection of aPL.

Antiphospholipid syndrome: laboratory diagnosis

Laboratory diagnosis of APS relies on the demonstration of a positive aCL antibody test by an in-house or commercially available enzyme-linked immunosorbent assay (ELISA) or on the presence of LA by a coagulation-based test. aCL should be tested in a β-2 glycoprotein I (β2-GPI)-dependent manner and LA should be diagnosed according to the International Society on Thrombosis and Haemostasis criteria [10–12].

Anticardiolipin antibodies

The aCL test is positive in about 80% of patients with APS, the LA test is positive in about 20%, and both are positive in about 60% of cases [13]. It is important that both tests be performed in patients suspected of having APS.

Although a sensitive test, aCL can be positive in a variety of disorders, including connective tissue diseases and infectious disorders such as syphilis [14,15], Q fever [16], and AIDS [17]. However, in these conditions, the predominant isotype is usually of the IgM class, present in low titers, and generally not associated with thrombotic features.

aCL have been shown to be a risk factor for first deep venous thrombosis [18] and recurrent venous thrombosis [19]. In a large prospective study of 360 unselected patients with LA with or without aCL, Finazzi and colleagues [20] showed that aCL above 40 GPL in patients with previous thrombotic events were independent predictors of subsequent vascular thrombosis. Other studies also found GPL titers to be important in identifying a higher risk group of patients for subsequent thrombo-occlusive events [21,22], although other studies have disagreed [23,24]. Their predictive value for arterial thrombosis and pregnancy morbidity in the general population is still to be defined.

Despite ongoing international efforts, interlaboratory agreement on aCL measurement is still low, mainly due to some methodologic and calibration issues. However, the use of a semiquantitative measure (ie, ranges of positivity low, medium, or high) seems to be adequate in most clinical settings and is less subject to error [25,26]. The use of a reliable, validated aCL ELISA kit may offer better reproducibility [26]. For in-house assays, calibrators derived from monoclonal antibodies, HCAL and EY2C9 [27] have been introduced in an effort to optimize standardization.

The observation that many aCL are directed to an epitope on β2GPI led to the development of the anti-β2GPI antibody (anti-β2GPI) immunoassay [28]. Anti-β2GPI are strongly associated with thrombosis and other features of APS [29]. Initial clinical studies of anti-β2GPI ELISAs suggest that positivity in these assays is more closely associated with aPL-related clinical manifestations than positivity in conventional aCL ELISAs [29]. As β2GPI-independent aCL usually does not correlate with thrombotic events, this may explain why anti-β2GPI ELISA is a more specific assay for the diagnosis of APS than aCL detected by conventional ELISA [30].

Anti-β2GPI assays have also identified a small number of patients who have clinical manifestations of the APS but are negative in conventional aPL assays [31].

Lupus anticoagulant

LA is identified by coagulation assays, in which it prolongs clotting times. A number of features need to be demonstrated: prolongation of a phospholipid-dependent clotting time; evidence of inhibition shown by mixing studies; evidence of phospholipid dependence; and exclusion of specific inhibition of any one coagulation factor. As they are very heterogeneous antibodies, it is necessary to perform more than one coagulation test to reach the diagnosis according to the classification criteria [11]. In principle, the laboratory tests to detect the LA should use a sensitive screening test followed by a specific confirmation test [12]. Both activated partial thromboplastin time and dilute Russell's viper venom time are suitable for testing LA [32,33]. However, in some subjects receiving oral anticoagulation, accurate detection of the LA might not be possible. In these cases, LA testing might be postponed until the patient is off anticoagulation, which is not sensible in most cases. Instead, patient sample can be diluted 1:2 with normal plasma (if international normalized ratio <3.5) before performing the tests [12,34]. Testing the Taipan or Textarin times might also be useful in these cases [12].

To satisfy classification criteria, the presence of aCL or LA should be detected on at least two occasions, 8 to 12 weeks apart [10,34]. Persistence of the positive tests must be demonstrated and other causes and underlying factors considered.

In general, LA are more specific than aCL for APS, although less sensitive. In general, there is a high concordance between LA and aCL [35–37], but these antibodies are not identical [38]. A meta-analysis evaluating the risk of venous thrombosis in SLE [39] showed that LA-positive subjects were six times more likely to have a thrombotic event than patients who were LA negative. Patients with aCL had a twofold increase in the risk of having a thrombotic event when compared with patients without aCL. These data were confirmed by a subsequent meta-analysis of aPL and venous thrombosis in patients without underlying immunologic disease that concluded that LA was a more specific predictor of thrombosis than aCL [40].

It has been demonstrated that patients with SLE are at a substantial risk of venous thrombosis over time. Both the presence of LA and polyclonal aCL are associated with the risk of venous thrombosis, although LA seems to be a better predictor of risk than aCL [41]. This has been confirmed in a recent systematic review of the literature where the LA was shown to be a risk factor for thrombosis, independent of the site (venous or arterial) and the type of the event (first or recurrence). In this analysis, aCL were not such strong risk factors, unless the IgG isotype and medium or high titers were considered [42].

Other antiphospholipid antibodies

The clinical utility of aPL antibody assays to phospholipids other than cardiolipin and to phospholipid-binding proteins other than β2GPI remains unclear [43]; the precise serologic "fingerprint" of the patients most at risk of thrombosis remains elusive [44].

Data on the clinical value of antibodies directed to prothrombin (another phospholipid binding protein) are contradictory. Antiprothrombin antibodies are heterogeneous, and can be directed to prothrombin coated onto irradiated plates (aPT) or to phosphatidylserine–prothrombin complex (aPS-PT) [45]. A recent systematic review showed no association between the presence of antiprothrombin antibodies and thrombosis, irrespective of isotype, site, and type of event and the presence of SLE [46]. In our experience, antiprothrombin antibodies are frequently found in SLE patients, and their presence is associated with APS [45]. Most significantly, some patients with aPL-related clinical features, who are negative for aCL, LA, and anti-β2GPI had antiprothrombin antibodies either by the aPT or the aPS-PT assays, suggesting that testing for these antibodies could be of clinical benefit in patients who are negative for the routine testing [45,47].

A number of other autoantibodies have been reported in patients with APS, including antibodies to annexin V [48,49], high and low molecular weight kininogens or, less frequently, prekallikrein and Factor XI [50,51]; to vascular heparan sulfate proteoglycan [52] heparin [53], factor XII [54–56], and thrombin [57]. Some data suggest that autoantibodies could be directed against components of protein C pathway [58], which includes protein C [59], protein S [60,61], and thrombomodulin [62]. The association of such antibodies with APS and their clinical significance is far from being known amid that these tests are far from standardized. Their application should be restricted only to research rather than to routine diagnostic use.

Which test should be used for the recognition of the antiphospholipid syndrome?

In 1998, a group of experts agreed by consensus that the two tests used in the recognition of APS should be the standardized β2-dependent aCL assay and the LA detected following the guidelines of the International Society for Thrombosis and Haemostasis [10]. Laboratory diagnosis of APS is based on a positive aCL antibody or LA test.

Although it cannot still be considered a replacement to aCL testing, a committee evaluating the new clinical, laboratory, and experimental insights since the 1999 publication of the Sapporo criteria considered to include IgG and IgM anti-β2GPI testing as a helpful diagnostic tool for the APS [34], particularly when aCL and LA are negative and APS is strongly suspected. However, due to the lack of standardization, their routine application still remains questionable. Laboratories around the world are being encouraged to solve these problems by standardizing the methodology applied and validating their measurements; the goal still has not been achieved.

A new assay that uses a mixture of negatively charged phospholipids has been proposed for more specific measurements of aPL [63]. The AphL phospholipid mixture was developed by testing aCL positive sera from a large number of patients with and without APS. A mixture able to discriminate APS from non-APS sera was identified [64]. A study examining this antigen suggests that the APhL ELISA kit may be a sensitive and relatively specific in identifying patients with APS [65].

Although new techniques for the detection of aPL, such as that detecting anti-β2GPI or antiprothrombin antibodies, have shown to be more specific than the aCL or LA [29,66], these tests are far from standardized. Moreover, one of the most important points to take into account is the lack of a universal positive or reference control. In these settings, the lack of agreement between laboratories (ie, source of the protein, type of ELISA plate, and so on) could highly influence the results obtained, making the application of these tests better restricted to research rather than to routine diagnostic use.

Seronegative antiphospholipid syndrome

This term was coined to characterize a group of patients with clinical manifestations of the APS, who are thought to have the syndrome despite negative results in conventional aPL testing (aCL or LA) [67,68]. Although it is universally recognized that the routine screening tests (aCL or LA) might miss some cases, careful differential diagnosis and repeat testing are mandatory before the diagnosis of "seronegative APS" can be made. This concept is important and certainly leaves room for further developments in testing for those autoantibodies that are thought to be associated with APS but not detected in conventional aPL assays.

Summary

Laboratory diagnosis of APS relies on the demonstration of a positive test for aPL. In clinical practice, the gold standard tests are those that detect β2GPI-dependent aCL or LA. The question on the use of anti-β2GPI as a routine diagnostic test remains unanswered, and testing for these antibodies should be only performed in very selected cases and not as an alternative to aCL or LA testing. Clinical utility and standardization are still lacking for other aPL specificities; therefore, their application as routine diagnostic tools is not recommended.

References

[1] Wasserman A, Neisser A, Bruck C. Eine serodiagnosticsche reaktion bei syphilis. Dtsch Med Wochenschr 1906;32:745–6.

[2] Pangborn MC. A new serologically active phospholipid from beef heart. Proc Soc Exp Biol Med 1941;48:484–6.

[3] Haserick JR, Long R. Systemic lupus erythematosus preceded by false-positive serologic test for syphilis: presentation of five cases. Ann Intern Med 1952;37:559–65.

[4] Conley CL, Hartmann RC. A hemorrhagic disorder caused by circulating anticoagulant in patients with disseminated lupus erythematosus. J Lab Clin Invest 1952;31:621–2.

[5] Beaumont JL. Syndrome hemorrhagique acquis du a un anticoagulant circulant. Sang 1954; 25:1–15.

[6] Laurell AB, Nilsson IM. Hypergammablobulinaemia, circulating anticoagulant and biological false positive Wasserman reaction: a study of 2 cases. J Lab Clin Med 1957;49:694–707.

[7] Bowie EJ, Thompson JKJ, Pascuzzi CA, et al. Thrombosis in systemic lupus erythematosus despite circulating anticoagulants. J Lab Clin Med 1963;62:416–30.

[8] Feinstein DI, Rapaport SI. Acquired inhibitors of blood coagulation. Prog Hemost Thromb 1972;1:75–95.

[9] Harris EN, Gharavi AE, Boey ML, et al. Anticardiolipin antibodies: detection by radioimmunoassay and association with thrombosis in systemic lupus erythematosus. Lancet 1983; ii(8361):1211–4.

[10] Wilson WA, Gharavi AE, Koike T, et al. International consensus statement on preliminary classification criteria for definite antiphospholipid syndrome: report of an international workshop. Arthritis Rheum 1999;42(7):1309–11.

[11] Brandt JT, Triplett DA, Alving B, et al. Criteria for the diagnosis of lupus anticoagulants: an update. On behalf of the Subcommittee on Lupus anticoagulant/Antiphospholipid Antibody of the Scientific and Standardisation Committee of the ISTH. Thromb Haemost 1995;74:1185–90.

[12] Greaves M, Cohen H, MacHin SJ, et al. Guidelines on the investigation and management of the antiphospholipid syndrome. Br J Haematol 2000;109(4):704–15.

[13] Cervera R, Piette JC, Font J, et al. Antiphospholipid syndrome: clinical and immunologic manifestations and patterns of disease expression in a cohort of 1,000 patients. Arthritis Rheum 2002;46(4):1019–27.

[14] Mouritsen S, Hoier-Madsen M, Wiik A, et al. The specificity of anti-cardiolipin antibodies from syphilis patients and from patients with systemic lupus erythematosus. Clin Exp Immunol 1989;76(2):178–83.

[15] Harris EN, Gharavi AE, Wasley GD, et al. Use of an enzyme-linked immunosorbent assay and of inhibition studies to distinguish between antibodies to cardiolipin from patients with syphilis or autoimmune disorders. J Infect Dis 1988;157(1):23–31.

[16] Galvez J, Martin I, Merino D, et al. Thrombophlebitis in a patient with acute Q fever and anticardiolipin antibodies. Med Clin (Barc) 1997;108(10):396–7.

[17] Intrator L, Oksenhendler E, Desforges L, et al. Anticardiolipin antibodies in HIV infected patients with or without immune thrombocytopenic purpura. Br J Haematol 1988;68(2): 269–70.

[18] Ginsburg KS, Liang MH, Newcomer L, et al. Anticardiolipin antibodies and the risk for ischemic stroke and venous thrombosis. Ann Intern Med 1992;117:997–1002.

[19] Schulman S, Svenungsson E, Granqvist S. Anticardiolipin antibodies predict early recurrence of thromboembolism and death among patients with venous thromboembolism following anticoagulant therapy. Duration of Anticoagulation Study Group. Am J Med 1998;104:332–8.

[20] Finazzi G, Brancaccio V, Moia M, et al. Natural history and risk factors for thrombosis in 360 patients with antiphospholipid antibodies: a four-year prospective study from the Italian Registry. Am J Med 1996;100(5):530–6.

[21] Escalante A, Brey RL, Mitchell BD Jr, et al. Accuracy of anticardiolipin antibodies in identifying a history of thrombosis among patients with systemic lupus erythematosus. Am J Med 1995;98(6):559–65.

[22] Levine SR, Salowich-Palm L, Sawaya KL, et al. IgG anticardiolipin antibody titer > 40 GPL and the risk of subsequent thrombo-occlusive events and death. A prospective cohort study. Stroke 1997;28(9):1660–5.

[23] Naess IA, Christiansen SC, Cannegieter SC, et al. A prospective study of anticardiolipin antibodies as a risk factor for venous thrombosis in a general population (the HUNT study). J Thromb Haemost 2006;4(1):44–9.

[24] Runchey SS, Folsom AR, Tsai MY, et al. Anticardiolipin antibodies as a risk factor for venous thromboembolism in a population-based prospective study. Br J Haematol 2002; 119(4):1005–10.

[25] Tincani A, Allegri F, Sanmarco M, et al. Anticardiolipin antibody assay: a methodological analysis for a better consensus in routine determinations—a cooperative project of the European Antiphospholipid Forum. Thromb Haemost 2001;86(2):575–83.

[26] Harris EN, Pierangeli SS. Revisiting the anticardiolipin test and its standardization. Lupus 2002;11(5):269–75.

[27] Ichikawa K, Tsutsumi A, Atsumi T, et al. A chimeric antibody with the human gamma1 constant region as a putative standard for assays to detect IgG beta2-glycoprotein I-dependent anticardiolipin and anti-beta2-glycoprotein I antibodies. Arthritis Rheum 1999;42(11): 2461–70.

[28] Matsuura E, Igarashi Y, Yasuda T, et al. Anticardiolipin antibodies recognize beta 2-glycoprotein I structure altered by interacting with an oxygen modified solid phase surface. J Exp Med 1994;179(2):457–62.

[29] Amengual O, Atsumi T, Khamashta MA, et al. Specificity of ELISA for antibody to beta 2-glycoprotein I in patients with antiphospholipid syndrome. Br J Rheumatol 1996;35(12): 1239–43.

[30] Balestrieri G, Tincani A, Spatola L, et al. Anti-beta 2-glycoprotein I antibodies: a marker of antiphospholipid syndrome? Lupus 1995;4(2):122–30.

[31] Cabral AR, Amigo MC, Cabiedes J, et al. The antiphospholipid/cofactor syndrome: a primary variant with antibodies to β2 glycoprotein I but no antibodies detectable in standard antiphospholipid assay. Am J Med 1996;101:472–81.

[32] Arnout J, Meijer P, Vermylen J. Lupus anticoagulant testing in Europe: an analysis of results from the first European Concerted Action on Thrombophilia (ECAT) survey using plasmas spiked with monoclonal antibodies against human beta2-glycoprotein I. Thromb Haemost 1999;81(6):929–34.

[33] Gardiner C, MacKie IJ, Malia RG, et al. The importance of locally derived reference ranges and standardized calculation of dilute Russell's viper venom time results in screening for lupus anticoagulant. Br J Haematol 2000;111(4):1230–5.

[34] Miyakis S, Lockshin MD, Atsumi T, et al. International consensus statement on an update of the classification criteria for definite antiphospholipid syndrome (APS). J Thromb Haemost 2006;4(2):295–306.

[35] Pengo V, Thiagarajan P, Shapiro SS, et al. Immunological specificity and mechanism of action of IgG lupus anticoagulants. Blood 1987;70(1):69–76.

[36] Galli M, Bevers EM, Comfurius P, et al. Effect of antiphospholipid antibodies on procoagulant activity of activated platelets and platelet-derived microvesicles. Br J Haematol 1993; 83(3):466–72.

[37] Triplett DA, Brandt JT, Musgrave KA, et al. The relationship between lupus anticoagulants and antibodies to phospholipid. JAMA 1988;259:550–4.

[38] McNeil HP, Chesterman CN, Krilis SA. Anticardiolipin antibodies and lupus anticoagulants comprise separate antibody subgroups with different phospholipid binding characteristics. Br J Haematol 1989;73(4):506–13.

[39] Wahl DG, Guillemin F, de Maistre E, et al. Risk for venous thrombosis related to antiphospholipid antibodies in systemic lupus erythematosus—a meta-analysis. Lupus 1997;6(5): 467–73.

[40] Wahl DG, Guillemin F, de Maistre E, et al. Meta-analysis of the risk of venous thrombosis in individuals with antiphospholipid antibodies without underlying autoimmune disease or previous thrombosis. Lupus 1998;7(1):15–22.

[41] Somers E, Magder LS, Petri M. Antiphospholipid antibodies and incidence of venous thrombosis in a cohort of patients with systemic lupus erythematosus. J Rheumatol 2002; 29(12):2531–6.

[42] Galli M, Luciani D, Bertolini G, et al. Lupus anticoagulants are stronger risk factors for thrombosis than anticardiolipin antibodies in the antiphospholipid syndrome: a systematic review of the literature. Blood 2003;101(5):1827–32.

[43] Levine JS, Branch DW, Rauch J. The antiphospholipid syndrome. N Engl J Med 2002; 346(10):752–63.

[44] Hughes GR. Migraine, memory loss, and "multiple sclerosis." Neurological features of the antiphospholipid (Hughes') syndrome. Postgrad Med J 2003;79(928):81–3.

[45] Bertolaccini ML, Atsumi T, Koike T, et al. Antiprothrombin antibodies detected in two different assay systems. Prevalence and clinical significance in systemic lupus erythematosus. Thromb Haemost 2005;93(2):289–97.

[46] Galli M, Luciani D, Bertolini G, et al. Anti-beta 2-glycoprotein I, antiprothrombin antibodies, and the risk of thrombosis in the antiphospholipid syndrome. Blood 2003;102(8): 2717–23.

[47] Bertolaccini ML, Gomez S, Pareja JF, et al. Antiphospholipid antibody tests: spreading the net. Ann Rheum Dis 2005;64(11):1639–43.

[48] Kaburaki J, Kuwana M, Yamamoto M, et al. Clinical significance of anti-annexin antibodies in patients with systemic lupus erythematosus. Am J Haematol 1997;54:209–13.

[49] Rand JH, Wu XX, Andree HAM, et al. Pregnancy loss in the antiphospholipid antibody syndrome—a possible thrombogenic mechanism. N Engl J Med 1997;337:154–60.

[50] Sugi T, McIntyre JA. Autoantibodies to phosphatidylethanolamine (PE) recognize a kininogen–PE complex. Blood 1995;86:3083–9.

[51] Sugi T, McIntyre JA. Certain autoantibodies to phosphatidylethanolamine (aPE) recognize Factor XI and Prekallikrein independently or in addition to the kininogens. J Autoimmun 2001;17:207–14.

[52] Shibata S, Harpel PC, Sasaki T, et al. Autoantibodies to vascular heparan sulfate proteoglycan in systemic lupus erythematosus react with endothelial cells and inhibit the formation of thrombin–antithrombin III complexes. Clin Immunol Immunopathol 1994;70: 114–23.

[53] Shibata S, Harpel PC, Gharavi A, et al. Autoantibodies to heparin from patients with antiphospholipid antibody syndrome inhibit formation of antithrombin III complexes. Blood 1994;83:2532–40.

[54] Jones DW, Gallimore MJ, Harris SL, et al. Antibodies to factor XII associated with lupus anticoagulant. Thromb Haemost 1999;81:387–90.

[55] Jones DW, Gallimore MJ, MacKie IJ, et al. Reduced factor XII levels in patients with the antiphospholipid syndrome are associated with antibodies to factor XII. Br J Haematol 2000;110:721–6.

[56] Jones DW, MacKie IJ, Gallimore MJ, et al. Antibodies to factor XII and recurrent fetal loss in patients with the anti-phospholipid syndrome. Br J Haematol 2001;113:550–2.

[57] Hwang KK, Grossman JM, Visvanathan S, et al. Identification of anti-thrombin antibodies in the antiphospholipid syndrome that interfere with the inactivation of thrombin by anti-thrombin. J Immunol 2001;167:7192–8.

[58] Oosting JD, Derksen RH, Bobbink IW, et al. Antiphospholipid antibodies directed against a combination of phospholipids with prothrombin, protein C, or protein S: an explanation for their pathogenic mechanism? Blood 1993;81(10):2618–25.

[59] Atsumi T, Khamashta MA, Amengual O, et al. Binding of anticardiolipin antibodies to protein C via beta2-glycoprotein I (beta2-GPI): a possible mechanism in the inhibitory effect of antiphospholipid antibodies on the protein C system. Clin Exp Immunol 1998;112(2):325–33.

[60] Erkan D, Zhang HW, Shriky RC, et al. Dual antibody reactivity to β2-glycoprotein I and Protein S: increased association with thrombotic events in the antiphospholipid syndrome. Lupus 2002;11(4):215–20.

[61] Bertolaccini ML, Sanna G, Ralhan S, et al. Antibodies directed to protein S in patients with systemic lupus erythematosus: prevalence and clinical significance. Thromb Haemost 2003; 90(4):636–41.

[62] Carson CW, Comp PC, Esmon NL, et al. Thrombomodulin antibodies inhibit protein C activation and are found in patients with lupus anticoagulant and unexplained thrombosis. Arthritis Rheum 1994;37:S296 [abstract].

[63] Pierangeli SS, Gharavi AE, Harris EN. Testing for antiphospholipid antibodies: problems and solutions. Clin Obstet Gynecol 2001;44(1):48–57.

[64] Pierangeli SS. Anticardiolipin testing. In: Khamashta MA, editor. Hughes syndrome. Antiphospholipid syndrome. 2nd ed. London: Springer-Verlag London Ltd; 2006. p. 275–90.

[65] Merkel PA, Chang Y, Pierangeli SS, et al. Comparison between the standard anticardiolipin antibody test and a new phospholipid test in patients with connective tissue diseases. J Rheumatol 1999;26(3):591–6.

[66] Atsumi T, Ieko M, Bertolaccini ML, et al. Association of autoantibodies against the phosphatidylserine–prothrombin complex with manifestations of the antiphospholipid syndrome and with the presence of lupus anticoagulant. Arthritis Rheum 2000;43(9):1982–93.

[67] Hughes GR, Khamashta MA. Seronegative antiphospholipid syndrome. Ann Rheum Dis 2003;62(12):1127.

[68] Roubey RAS. Antiphospholipid syndrome in the absence of standard antiphospholipid antibodies: associations with other autoantibodies. In: Khamashta MA, editor. Hughes syndrome. Antiphospholipid syndrome. 2nd ed. London: Springer-Verlag London Ltd; 2006. p. 329–37.

ELSEVIER
SAUNDERS

Rheum Dis Clin N Am
32 (2006) 465–490

RHEUMATIC
DISEASE CLINICS
OF NORTH AMERICA

Cerebral Manifestations in the Antiphospholipid (Hughes) Syndrome

Giovanni Sanna, MD, FRCP, PhD[a],*,
David D'Cruz, MD, FRCP[b],
Maria Jose Cuadrado, MD, PhD[b]

[a]*Department of Rheumatology, Homerton University Hospital,
London E9 6SR, United Kingdom*
[b]*Louise Coote Lupus Unit, St. Thomas' Hospital, London SE1 7EH, United Kingdom*

The antiphospholipid (Hughes) syndrome (APS), the most frequent type of acquired thrombophilia, is defined by the occurrence of thrombosis or pregnancy morbidity in the presence of persistently positive anticardiolipin antibodies (aCL) or lupus anticoagulant (LA) [1,2]. A large variety of clinical manifestations including arterial and venous thrombosis in large and small vessels, obstetric complications, skin disease, cardiac and pulmonary features, renal involvement, hematologic manifestations, and neurologic disorders can be seen in patients with APS [3,4].

Twenty-three years since its original description, the major impact of APS on neurology is now largely recognized [5]. Cerebral involvement in APS is common, and results in different clinical manifestations [6]. The importance of neurologic features was indeed foreseen in the original description of the syndrome by Graham Hughes [7] and in the early 1980s, when his group reported the association of antiphospholipid antibodies (aPL) with a wide spectrum of neuropsychiatric manifestations including cerebral ischemia, dementia, migraine, seizures, chorea, transverse myelitis, and Guillain-Barré syndrome [8–11].

A large number of other neuropsychiatric features, including chronic headache, cognitive dysfunction, psychosis, depression, and multiple sclerosis-like disease have also been described in association with aPL [6,12–16]. The spectrum of cerebral manifestations associated with aPL is summarized in Box 1.

* Corresponding author.
  E-mail address: giovanni.sanna@homerton.nhs.uk (G. Sanna).

0889-857X/06/$ - see front matter © 2006 Elsevier Inc. All rights reserved.
doi:10.1016/j.rdc.2006.05.010

rheumatic.theclinics.com

Box 1. Clinical classification of neuropsychiatric manifestations associated with the presence of antiphospholipid antibodies

Focal neurologic manifestations
Cerebrovascular disease
   Transient ischemic attacks
   Ischemic stroke
   Sneddon's syndrome
   Acute ischemic encephalopathy
   Moyamoya disease
   Cerebral venous thrombosis
Seizures (partial)
Migraine
Movement disorders
   Chorea
   Dystonia-Parkinsonism
Multiple sclerosis like-syndrome
Myelopathy
Idiopathic intracranial hypertension
Other neurologic syndromes
   Sensorineural hearing loss
   Ocular syndromes
   Transient global amnesia
   Guillain-Barré syndrome

Diffuse neuropsychiatric manifestations
Generalized seizures
Headache (other than migraine)
Cognitive dysfunction
Dementia
Other psychiatric disorders
   Depression
   Psychosis

Pathogenesis

The mechanism of cerebral involvement in APS is considered to be primarily thrombotic. However, pathogenesis is not completely understood. Although there is some evidence that cerebral endothelium may be activated by aPL with promotion of procoagulant activity [17–20], it is not clear how these antibodies initiate thrombosis [21]. There is also evidence that aPL may bind glial cells, myelin, and neurons, disrupting their function with direct pathogenetic effects [22–24]. It has recently been suggested that aPL may play a direct role in causing cognitive and behavioral impairments

[25], and animal models are providing important insights into some of the underlying mechanisms for this type of central nervous sytems (CNS) dysfunction [26,27]. It is possible that the prothrombotic state associated with aPL is responsible for alterations of the cerebral microcirculation as the underlying cause for some type of diffuse neuropsychiatric manifestations observed in APS, including seizures and cognitive dysfunction. Ziporen and colleagues [28] have recently shown that thrombotic occlusion of capillaries with mild inflammation may underlie the neurologic defects displayed in a mouse model of APS.

Clinical features

Cerebrovascular disease

The most common serious complication and cause of significant morbidity in APS is stroke. It has been suggested that up to one in five of all strokes in young people (under 45) strokes may be associated with APS [14]. Several studies have shown that strokes and transient ischemic attacks (TIAs) are the commonest arterial thrombotic event in patients with APS [3,29–31]. Stroke patients with aPL are younger and more likely to be women in comparison with stroke patients without aPL [32,33]. Amaurosis fugax, transient paresthesias, ataxia, motor weakness, vertigo, and transient global ischemia can all be expressions of TIAs [34].

Early studies suggested that left-sided valve vegetations can be a source for emboli and a possible cause of ischemic stroke in aPL patients [35–37]. Khamashta and colleagues [38] showed that the prevalence of valvular abnormalities is higher in systemic lupus erythematosus (SLE) patients with aPL than in those without. More recently, Krause and colleagues [39] reported on a close association between valvular heart disease and several CNS manifestations—not only stroke and TIA, but also epilepsy and migraine—in a large group of APS patients, supporting early observations of valve lesions as a possible risk factor for cerebral emboli in these patients.

The presence of aPL is strongly associated with stroke and TIAs in SLE patients. We recently found cerebrovascular disease in 14.5% of 323 consecutive SLE patients and confirmed a strong association between the presence of aPL and cerebrovascular disease in SLE [40].

Many studies have found that aPL are associated with an increased risk for cerebral ischemia in the general population [41–52], although some have not [53–57].

Brey and colleagues [50] found an association between aPL and stroke over a 20-year period of follow-up in men enrolled in the Honolulu Heart program, with the presence of β2GPI-dependent aCL of the IgG isotype significantly associated with both incident ischemic stroke and myocardial infarction. Janardhan and colleagues [52] recently published the results of a large prospective population-based cohort study with an 11-year period of follow-up in the context of the Framingham Heart Study. They showed that aCL are an independent risk factor for ischemic stroke and TIA in women after multivariate adjustment for other cardiovascular risk factors.

However, it is still controversial whether the presence of aPL at the time of initial stroke increases the risk of recurrence in an unselected population. In 1997, Levine and colleagues [58] showed that the risk for recurrent stroke was higher in patients with aPL after the first cerebral ischemic episode. These results were not confirmed in two studies by the Antiphospholipid Antibodies and Stroke Study (APASS) Group [59,60]. Levine and the APASS investigators [60] recently reported that the presence of either LA or aCL among patients with ischemic stroke did not predict an increased risk for further thrombo-occlusive events. The authors concluded that routine screening for aPL did not appear warranted in patients with ischemic stroke. A number of important limitations of this study have raised several concerns [61–64]: (1) the average age of patients (62.5 years) was significantly higher than in previous studies of APS (34 years) [3]; (2) only a single measurement of aCL and LA was obtained; (3) a high proportion of patients was found positive for aPL (41%), but only 0.2% had high IgG levels, and only 6.7% tested positive for both aCL and LA. Interestingly, the group of patients positive for both aCL and LA had a tendency to develop recurrent events. Although this recent study doubted whether the presence of aPL increases the risk of recurrent stroke or other thromboembolic events, most data point to persistent medium/high titer aCL or LA as a major risk factor for recurrence. A recent systematic review of the literature showed LA to be a risk factor for thrombosis, independent of the site (venous or arterial) and the type of event (first or recurrence). aCL were not such strong risk factors, unless the IgG isotype and medium and high titers were considered [65].

Another recent study failed to find a higher incidence of recurrent cerebral ischemia in children positive for aPL [66]. This study included 185 children surviving a first ischemic stroke or TIA who were tested for aCL and followed for a median of 2.8 years. Although a higher rate of recurrent arterial ischemic stroke/TIA was observed (36%), no differences were found in rates of recurrent thromboembolism between aCL positive and aCL-negative groups. The main limitation of this study is the fact that aCL-positive children were more likely to be treated with antithrombotic agents than those negative for aCL. Those receiving treatment had, in turn, a reduced risk of recurrent ischemic stroke or TIA.

Sneddon's syndrome

Sneddon's syndrome is defined by the development of cerebrovascular disease (stroke or TIA) in the presence of widespread livedo reticularis. The predominant pathology is a noninflammatory occlusive arteriopathy [67] in this condition that mainly affects women before or during middle age. The pathogenesis of Sneddon's syndrome has remained largely unclear since Sneddon's original description of four cases in 1965 [68].

Some authors have suggested including this condition among the neurologic manifestations of APS [69–72]. There have been an increasing number of reports of an association of Sneddon's syndrome with aPL [73]. Frances and colleagues [74] found a prevalence of aPL of around 41% in patients diagnosed with Sneddon's syndrome, and Kalashnikova and colleagues [75] reported more severe progression of the neurologic disease in patients with Sneddon's syndrome and high levels of aCL. Recently Gomez-Puerta and colleagues [16] confirmed these observations in their study of the clinical and radiologic characteristics of dementia associated with APS. They found that 10 of 30 patients (33%) with APS and dementia also had Sneddon's syndrome.

On the other hand, livedo reticularis is a frequent cutaneous manifestation in patients with APS. In a recent study Toubi and colleagues [76] found livedo reticularis in 16% of 308 APS patients. Interestingly enough, they also found a strong association with cerebrovascular disease, migraines, epilepsy, cardiac valve thickening, and vegetations, suggesting that patients with APS and livedo reticularis are at higher risk for thrombosis.

Sneddon's syndrome is not a unique entity, and aPL may play a pathogenic role in a subset of patients with this disorder. It is possible that some patients diagnosed as having Sneddon's syndrome actually have APS. The distinction is important as the treatment of APS (ie, anticoagulation) differs from that of Sneddon's syndrome.

Less common types of cerebrovascular disease

Acute ischemic encephalopathy has been found in only 1.1% of APS patients in the cohort of the Euro-Phospholipid Project Group study, the largest cohort described to date [3]. This rare neurologic manifestation was first found in association with aPL in 1989 [77]. Patients with acute ischemic encephalopathy present acutely ill, confused, and disoriented. The most frequent finding on MRI is cerebral atrophy.

There are a few reports of an association of aPL with moyamoya disease, a rare disorder of uncertain cause characterized by progressive vascular stenosis and blockage of the cerebral arteries [78–83]. The name moyamoya comes from the Japanese, and it means "puff of smoke," which is the description of the angiographic appearance of the collateral circulation due to the vascular blockage. This condition tends to affect children under 10 years of age, and has rarely been described in adults (3–4 decade). The association between APS and moyamoya disease has been reported only in children so far [83]. These young patients may present clinically with seizures, TIA, or stroke. Booth and colleagues [80] reported on a 7-year-old with ischemic stroke and persistently raised levels of aCL in the presence of moyamoya-like vascular changes. Treatment with warfarin and aspirin was followed by improvement in blood flow and reduction in the stenosis of the left internal carotid artery. Recently, Yamashita and colleagues [83] reported on a 12-year-old Japanese female who presented with choreic movements and thrombocytopenia, persistently positive aCL and LA, and typical angiographic features of moyamoya disease.

Venous sinus thrombosis, a rare form of cerebral thrombotic disease, generally occurs at a younger age and with more extensive superficial and deep cerebral venous system involvement in patients with aPL than in those without [84–89]. In these patients aPL are often present in association with other concomitant risk factors for thrombophilia [90]. These patients may present clinically with headache, nausea, vomiting, impairment of consciousness, and papilloedema. MRI is very helpful to confirm the diagnosis. The prevalence of cerebral venous thrombosis was 0.7% in the Euro-Phospholipid cohort [3].

Seizures

A number of studies [40,91–96] have confirmed early observations [97,98] of the association between aPL and seizures. The increased prevalence of autoantibodies in patients with epilepsy has been attributed to the use of antiepileptic drugs [99]. However, recent studies showed no associations between the presence of autoantibodies, including aPL, and antiepileptic medications in patients with epilepsy [93,100–102]. Generalized tonic–clonic seizures are the most common, but simple partial and complex seizures have also been described in association with aPL [40,96].

The majority of the studies regarding epilepsy are related to SLE or to APS associated to SLE, and few data have been produced regarding epilepsy in primary APS. Cervera and colleagues [3] reported seizures in 7% of 1000 patients with APS. More recently, Shoenfeld and colleagues [15] reported epilepsy with a prevalence of 8.6% in a cohort of 538 patients with APS. They found that epilepsy was more frequent in patients with secondary APS (13.7%) than in those with primary APS (6%), and that patients with epilepsy had a higher prevalence of focal ischemic events. Appenzeller and colleagues [96] recently observed seizures in 11.6% of 519 SLE patients. Stroke and moderate–high titers of IgG aCL were associated with seizures at disease onset. Patients with renal flares, seizures at disease onset, and positive aPL were at greater risk for seizures during follow-up, and recurrent seizures were observed in seven patients, all of them with APS. Seizures are a well-known symptom of cerebral ischemia [103], and it is possible that in many cases seizures are caused by ischemic events in aPL patients. However, this explains only part of the increased frequency of epilepsy in APS, and a primary immunologic basis for seizures in APS has also been postulated. There is evidence of a direct effect of aPL on neuronal tissue as a possible alternative mechanism to hypercoagulability [24,104,105]. It has been shown that aCL from patients with SLE with seizures reduce a gamma-aminobutyric acid (GABA) receptor-mediated chloride current in snail neurons [104], and that aPL may lower the seizure threshold with a direct (and reversible) mechanism. It has been shown that aPL may bind directly to ependyma and myelin of fixed cat [106] and rat brains [107], and that aPL depolarize brain nerve terminals [105]. Although the pathogenetic mechanisms underlying the association of seizures with aPL remain uncertain, it is possible that these antibodies play a role at least in certain types of seizures and different clinical studies support this hypothesis. A recent article from Ranua and colleagues [102] found an association between a long duration of partial epilepsy and poor seizure control (despite antiepileptic treatment) and the presence of aCL. In a previous study from our group, seizures were found to be associated with moderate-to-high titers of aCL [91]. Liou and colleagues [108] confirmed an association between epilepsy and high titers of aCL, with an odds ratio of developing seizures of 3.7 for SLE patients who had a high baseline serum level of aCL when compared with those without a detectable level of these antibodies. Our more recent study confirmed a strong association between the aPL and seizures in a large series of SLE patients [40]. We reported seizures in 8.3% of 323 patients with SLE. Both IgG and IgM aCL were more prevalent among patients with seizures when compared with those without. The association of seizures with aCL remained significant after excluding 47 patients with stroke or TIAs, and multivariate analysis confirmed that aCL were independently associated with cerebrovascular accidents and seizures. Another recent study by Mikdashi and Handwerger [109] supports the importance of aPL as an independent risk factor for seizures, cerebrovascular accidents, and cognitive impairment, as shown by others [40,110]. In a recently published paper, Lampropoulos and colleagues [111] found that abnormalities on electroencephalography are common in patients with APS, and correlate with the presence of aPL in patients with SLE even in the absence of abnormalities on MRI.

Headache and migraine

Chronic headaches, including migraines, are common in patients with APS [3,112]. The headaches are often intractable, unresponsive to narcotic analgesics, and can antedate the diagnosis by many years. Surprisingly, despite the overwhelmingly strong clinical association, the published data on the association of headaches with aPL is still controversial [113–115], and the exact prevalence of headaches in patients with APS is unknown. Several problems contribute to these differences, especially the use of different classifications for headaches in the different studies. The available data suggest no association between aPL and migraines. Montalban and colleagues [114] prospectively studied 103 patients with SLE and 58 patients with migraines without SLE. They found a high frequency of headaches in SLE patients, but no association of aCL with migraines. Similar negative results have been shown in other studies [116,117]. In our recent study in 323 SLE patients we found that although the prevalence of headaches was similar to that reported for the general population, aPL were more significantly prevalent in the group of patients with headaches compared with those without. However, we failed to find an association between the presence of aPL and any particular type of headache, including migraines [40]. On the other hand, numerous studies on the prevalence of aPL in migraine sufferers have failed to find any association [118–121]. Tietjen and colleagues [115] assessed the frequency of aCL in migraines in a prospective study including large different groups of patients: 645 patients had transient focal neurologic events, 518 migraines with aura, 497 migraines without aura, and 366 were healthy controls. They failed to find any association between aCL and migraines. There is only one study [122] that found a higher prevalence of aCL in 65 migraine patients, but the study was not controlled and the number of patients was small. Verrotti and colleagues [123] found no association between aCL and migraines in children in a prospective study. In summary, to date, prospective, controlled studies have failed to demonstrate an association between aPL and migraines in SLE patients or a higher prevalence of aPL in migraine sufferers.

Chorea and other movement disorders

Chorea is a rare manifestation, with an estimated prevalence of 1.3% in patients with APS [3]. Although rare, chorea has been strongly associated with the presence of aPL from the earliest descriptions of the syndrome [124,125]. The etiology of chorea is still unknown. Because chorea is often unilateral, acute in onset, and often followed by other CNS manifestations, a vascular pathogenesis has been postulated. However, in many patients with chorea, focal lesions on brain imaging have often been absent [124,125], casting doubt on a purely thrombotic cause. It has been suggested that aPL can cause chorea by directly binding phospholipid in the basal ganglia as a possible alternative mechanism to hypercoagulability [126]. Cervera and colleagues [127] reviewed the clinical, radiologic, and immunologic characteristics of 50 patients with chorea and APS. Fifty-eight percent of patients had defined SLE, 12% "lupus-like" syndrome, 30% had primary APS. Twelve percent of patients developed chorea soon after they started taking estrogen-containing oral contraceptives, 6% developed chorea gravidarum, and 2% of patients developed chorea shortly after delivery. Most patients (66%) had only one episode of chorea. Chorea was bilateral in 55% of patients. Computed tomography and MRI scans reported cerebral infarcts in 35% of patients.

There are a few anecdotal reports of Parkinsonism in association with APS [128,129]. Milanov and colleagues [129] recently reported on the combination of dystonia with Parkinsonian-like symptoms as a presenting clinical manifestation of APS in a 60-year-old man who had ischemic lesions in the basal ganglia on MRI and positive aPL. Reiblat and colleagues [130] recently reported on a 52-year-old man with Parkinson's disease who developed severe headache, progressive dementia, ataxia, downgaze palsy, and axial and limb rigidity. Treatment with levodopa was introduced without any improvement in his condition, and the diagnosis was modified to supranuclear palsy. Subsequently, he developed livedo reticularis and thrombocytopenia with positive aCL and LA. It has been suggested that anticoagulation should be considered in patients with aPL and dystonia-Parkinsonism to prevent further deterioration in case of lack of clinical improvement with levodopa, bromocriptine, and anticholinergics [131].

Multiple sclerosis-like syndrome

Clinical syndromes mimicking multiple sclerosis (MS), mainly in its relapsing-remitting pattern, are reported to occur in association with aPL [12,132,133]. In the majority of cases it is not difficult to differentiate between APS and MS. The difficulty only lies in the rare atypical cases, which may represent a diagnostic dilemma. Some APS patients can be misdiagnosed as having MS, making this a crucial point for the therapeutic approach [14]. There are no definite diagnostic tests for MS and APS. Analysis of the oligoclonal bands is not specific for MS, and the finding of positive aPL is not specific for APS. A few studies found a variable prevalence of aPL, ranging from 8 to 33%, in MS patients, in the absence of clinical features of systemic autoimmunity or APS [134–136]. In selected cases, changes in the white matter in APS patients may be difficult to differentiate from those of MS, making the differential diagnosis extremely difficult. In a study from our unit, we analyzed 27 APS patients in whom an original diagnosis of MS was made, in an attempt to identify parameters that might differentiate the two entities. Neurologic symptoms and physical examination of the patients were not different from those common in MS patients. A careful medical history, a previous history of thrombosis, or pregnancy morbidity in female patients may contribute to help in the differential diagnosis, favoring APS [12,14]. A recent cross-sectional study by Figved and colleagues [137] showed that the most common neuropsychiatric symptom in MS patients is depression, in keeping with previous studies [138,139]. Therefore, the abruptness of onset and resolution of symptoms, especially in regard to visual symptoms (ie, amaurosis fugax), and atypical neurologic features for MS such as headache or epilepsy, suggest APS rather than MS [140]. In the majority of the patients ultimately correctly diagnosed with APS and appropriately anticoagulated, there were no further neurologic events [14]. We think that if not all, at least a subgroup of patients with "nonclassical" MS should be tested for aPL. Paran and colleagues [141] recently showed that abnormal evoked potential studies are more prevalent in patients with MS than in those with APS. They studied 30 patients with APS and 33 patients with definite MS of similar neurologic disability and found abnormal visual evoked potential in 58% of MS patients and in 10% of APS ($P = 0.0005$), and abnormal upper limb somatosensory evoked potential in 33% of MS and 6% of APS ($P = 0.008$). The finding of normal evoked potentials may therefore favor the possibility of APS and be helpful in particular difficult cases in differentiating between the two conditions.

Myelopathy

This is a rare manifestation, with a recently estimated prevalence of less than 1% in patients with APS [3,142]. There is a strong association between transverse myelitis in SLE and the presence of aPL. In 1985, Harris and colleagues [10] first reported on a case of transverse myelitis associated with aPL in their description of a 45-year-old woman with a lupus-like illness and high titer positivity for aCL. Other authors confirmed this initial observation. Alarcon-Segovia and colleagues [143] found a higher prevalence of aPL in SLE patients with transverse myelitis than in those without, and subsequently, Lavalle and colleagues [144] reported on 10 of 12 SLE patients with transverse myelitis who tested positive for aCL, and the other 2 with evidence of a Venereal Disease Research Laboratory-positive test and prolonged activated partial thromboplastin time. Kovacs and colleagues [145] evaluated 14 patients with SLE and transverse myelitis and 91 additional cases published in the literature. Forty three percent of their patients and 64% of the patients reported in the literature were aPL positive. More recently, D'Cruz and colleagues [146] described a series of 15 patients with transverse myelitis as the presenting manifestation of SLE or lupus-like disease. Interestingly, 73% of the patients were aPL positive, supporting the view of a strong association of transverse myelitis with aPL. The pathophysiology of spinal cord damage in aPL-associated myelopathy is uncertain; however, both ischemia and antibody-mediated interaction have been postulated.

Idiopathic intracranial hypertension

Idiopathic intracranial hypertension can be the presenting symptom of APS, and the available evidence supports the hypothesis that aPL may play a role in the pathogenesis of this manifestation. However, the true incidence of idiopathic intracranial hypertension in APS patients is still unknown. Following a few anecdotal reports on the presence of aPL in patients with idiopathic intracranial hypertension [147,148], more recent studies confirmed that these antibodies are strongly associated with this neurologic complication. Sussman and colleagues [149] found that a substantial number of patients with intracranial hypertension were positive for aCL (11 of 38, 29%), but only four of them had aCL without evidence of underlying sinus thrombosis or any other associated prothrombotic risk factor. More interesting were the findings of Leker and colleagues [150], who found persistently elevated titers of aCL in 6 out of 14 patients (43%) with idiopathic intracranial hypertension. The association between aPL and idiopathic intracranial hypertension was more recently confirmed by Kesler and colleagues [151] in a retrospective study.

Other neurologic syndromes

Sensorineural hearing loss

The association between sensorineural hearing loss and aPL, initially reported anecdotally [152–154], has recently been confirmed by several authors [155–157]. Toubi and colleagues [155] found that 27% of 30 patients with sudden sensorineural hearing loss were positive for aCL compared with 0% of the control group, suggesting that aPL may play a primary role in the pathogenesis of this condition. Naarendorp and colleagues [156] also described six patients with SLE or a lupus-like syndrome, who developed sudden sensorineural hearing loss and had elevated serum levels of aCL or positivity for LA. More recently, Green and Miller [157] described a case of sudden sensorineural hearing loss in association with aPL as a first manifestation of SLE, and suggested anticoagulant treatment for these patients.

Guillain-Barré syndrome

Guillain-Barré syndrome is a transient neurologic disorder characterized by an inflammatory demyelination of peripheral nerves. Although the pathogenesis of this disorder has not been elucidated, there is increasing evidence pointing to an autoimmune etiology. This demyelinating neuropathy, also uncommon in SLE patients, was associated with aPL in the original descriptions of the Hughes syndrome [8]. Gilburd and colleagues [158] studied the reactivity of Guillain-Barré syndrome sera with various phospholipids, which are known to be important constituents of myelin, and serve as autoantigens in other autoimmune conditions, demonstrating that some Guillain-Barré syndrome patients produce autoantibodies to various phospholipid and nuclear antigens. However, these autoantibodies are probably produced as a result of the myelin damage rather than cause the demyelination.

Transient global amnesia

Transient global amnesia, a syndrome of sudden unexplained short-term memory loss in association with aPL, was reported by Montalban and colleagues [159]. Some regard this disturbance as migrainous in origin, but other mechanisms such as epileptic seizure have been advocated as involved in its pathogenesis [160].

Ocular syndromes

Ophthalmologic features are present in 15% to 88% of the patients with APS. An ophthalmic assessment should be part of the clinical evaluation of any patients with suspected or confirmed APS [161]. Amaurosis fugax suggests cerebral ischemia, and is one of the most common ocular manifestations in APS. Other visual disturbances have been associated with the presence of aPL. Ischemic optic neuropathy is less frequently described in APS when compared with SLE patients [162,163]. Frohman and colleagues [164] recently reported on the association between primary APS and autoimmune optic neuropathy in a 4-year-old child who presented four consecutive episodes of bilateral optic neuritis, one episode of unilateral optic neuritis, weakness, and ataxia in the presence of persistently raised aCL and abnormal skin biopsy showing microthrombosis. Papais-Alvarenga and colleagues [165] described clinical features and outcome of 24 Brazilian patients with optic neuromyelitis syndrome. Interestingly, three patients with recurrent optic neuropathy also had APS. Vasoocclusive retinopathy has also been described in the presence of aPL [166]. This is a rare but severe form of retinopathy characterized by microthrombosis and often associated with other CNS manifestations [167]. Poor visual outcome with visual loss has been reported in 80% of cases, with neovascularization occurring in 40% of cases [167]. aPL have also been noted in a patient with acute multifocal posterior placoid pigment epitheliopathy, a disorder that has been associated with retinal vascular occlusive disease [168].

Cognitive dysfunction

Cognitive dysfunction varies from global dysfunction in the context of multiinfarct dementia to subtle cognitive deficits in otherwise asymptomatic patients with aPL. One of the most common complaints in these patients is of poor memory, difficulty in concentrating, or difficulty in keeping their attention for a long time, indicating a possible preclinical phase of neurologic involvement. Most published data are related to SLE patients, with limited data regarding cognitive dysfunction in APS patients. In the largest published series of APS to date a prevalence of 2% was reported for multiinfarct dementia, but no data were provided on different types of cognitive dysfunction [3]. The recognition of subtle forms of cognitive dysfunction has been facilitated by the application of formal neuropsychologic assessment, mainly in patients with SLE [40,169–173].

The relationship of cognitive dysfunction with aPL has been investigated in cross-sectional [174,175] and prospective/longitudinal studies [176,177]. Verbal and nonverbal memory, including working memory, verbal fluency, psychomotor speed, and cognitive flexibility, and decreased overall productivity have been correlated with aPL [175–177]. In the studies from Menon and colleagues [177] and Hanly and colleagues [176], SLE patients persistently positive for aCL (medium to high titer) had significantly lower scores on a variety of neuropsychologic tests than SLE patients negative for aPL. There was no association between results of neuropsychologic tests and levels of anti-DNA or C3 fraction levels.

Denburg and colleagues [175] also found that LA-positive patients performed worse in measures of verbal memory, cognitive flexibility, and psychomotor speed. This pattern of deficits was compatible with a subcortical involvement, possibly on the basis of ongoing LA-related microthrombotic events or vasculopathy. Because many of these patients had no previous history of any neuropsychiatric involvement, the authors also suggested a direct relationship between the presence of aPL and cognitive impairment.

Whether these cognitive deficits are related to recurrent cerebral ischemia or whether there is any other underlying mechanism is not clear. It is possible that aPL play a more direct pathogenetic role in causing cognitive dysfunction, as shown by recent experimental studies. It has been demonstrated that aPL may gain access to the CNS [178], disrupt neuronal function [105], and play a direct role in the pathogenesis of behavioral impairment in animal models of APS [24,25,27,179].

The clinical implications of these findings are that, although the current evidence does not support the introduction of aggressive anticoagulation as a strategy to prevent subclinical cognitive impairment, there may be a role for more benign therapies such as low-dose aspirin or antimalarials. On the other hand, anecdotal reports of improvement of these symptoms after anticoagulation therapy commenced for other reasons in APS patients [180], may provide some support for the theory that arterial thrombosis or ischamia represent the primary cause of this type of CNS dysfunction, supporting the utility of further longitudinal case–control trials to answer the question of whether an anticoagulation treatment with low targeted international normalized ratio (INR) could be superior to aspirin in these patients.

Dementia

A chronic multifocal disease, defined as a recurrent or progressive neurologic deterioration attributable to cerebrovascular disease, can produce multiinfarct dementia. Dementia is an unusual manifestation of APS [3], but has a high disability impact in a patient's daily life. In 1989, Asherson and colleagues [34] described the clinical and serologic features of 35 patients with aPL and cerebrovascular disease. Strokes were often multiple, and were followed by multiinfarct dementia in nine patients. This dementia, generally associated with a loss of cognitive functions and impairment of skills, concentration, memory dysfunction, language impairment, and judgemental defects, does not present with specific characteristics. It cannot be differentiated from other kinds of dementia such as in Alzheimer's disease, senile dementia, or metabolic/toxic conditions involving the brain. Many other authors have since reported this complication in patients with recurrent strokes [181–183].

Mosek and colleagues [184] examined the relationship of aPL to dementia in the elderly in a case–controlled study. They found that 5 of the 87 demented patients (6%), but none of the 69 controls, had significantly elevated aCL IgG levels (above 20 GPL). All the patients with high aCL IgG levels were diagnosed clinically as having dementia of the Alzheimer type, except for one who had mixed dementia, and none had features of an immune-mediated disease. This study showed that a small but significant number of patients with dementia may have high levels of aPL. The role of the aPL in these patients, with apparently diffuse brain disease, is currently unknown. Chapman and colleagues [185] recently confirmed the association of APS with dementia in a hospital-based study. They found that 13 out of 23 patients (56%) with primary APS were demented. These patients were older and had higher levels of aPL when compared with the nondemented APS patients. The authors suggested that the length of exposure to aPL may play an important role—as well the presence of high levels of aPL—in determining the development of dementia. In a recent paper, Gomez-Puerta and colleagues [16] reviewed the characteristics of 30 patients (25 patients identified by a search of the literature and 5 from their clinical center) with dementia associated with APS. The mean age of patients was 49 ± 15 years. Forty-seven percent of patients had primary APS, 30% SLE, and 23% "lupus-like" syndrome. Thirty-seven percent of patients had cerebrovascular accidents, 33% cerebrovascular disease in association with livedo reticularis (Sneddon's syndrome), and 27% heart valve lesions. Although 63% of patients had APS manifestations before the diagnosis of dementia, only a minority (37%) were receiving anticoagulation. The mean time of evolution from the initial manifestation of APS to the diagnosis of dementia in these patients was 3.5 years. The authors recommended testing for aPL in young subjects with no explicable cause of dementia for the possibility of APS and appropriate antithrombotic prophylaxis once the diagnosis of APS is made to prevent disease progression.

Other psychiatric disorders

Psychiatric problems such as mood alterations and psychosis may be present in patients with APS, although both the frequency and the pathophysiologic relationship to APS remain controversial. It is also possible that these findings are complicated by the development in some cases of drug-induced aPL [186]. It is also difficult to establish whether or not the psychiatric symptoms are due to a psychologic reaction of suffering from a chronic disorder [187].

Brain imaging

Brain MRI in aPL patients with ischemic stroke typically shows cortical abnormalities consistent with large vessel occlusion. However, small high-density lesions on the brain MRI are frequently found in patients with aPL and, in our experience, also in SLE patients with or without overt neuropsychiatric manifestations [188]. The significance of widespread white matter hyperintensity lesions is not completely understood. It has been suggested that they may be due to multiple small infarcts. There is also evidence that the presence of similar lesions is associated with a higher risk for stroke [189], dementia, and cognitive decline in the elderly population [190]. The finding of white matter hyperintensities on the brain MRI may represent a diagnostic and therapeutic dilemma, especially when recognized in young patients. In our experience, subclinical cognitive disorders, usually undetected in the absence of a formal neuropsychologic assessment, are frequent in these patients. In a recent study we also found that small high-density lesions on the brain MRI were associated with the presence of LA [40], suggesting the possibility of an underlying ischemic/thrombotic mechanism for these lesions. A recent article by Steens and colleagues [191] also supports the hypothesis of a role of aPL in the pathogenesis of diffuse microscopic brain damage. In this preliminary study the authors evaluated the correlation between gray and white matter magnetization transfer ratio parameters and the presence of IgM and IgG aCL and LA in 18 patients with SLE with history of neuropsychiatric SLE but without cerebral infarcts on conventional MRI. They observed an association between lower values for mean magnetization transfer ratio and presence of aPL, suggesting that these antibodies may contribute to widespread microscopic brain damage in SLE patients. As recognized by the authors, the main limitations of this work were the small number of patients studied and the lack of a control group.

Abnormalities in regional cerebral blood flow by the SPECT study have been reported in APS patients [192–196]. Two recent studies [192,195] have reported brain SPECT abnormalities in patients with primary APS and mild diffuse neuropsychiatric manifestations (headache, memory loss, or other cognitive function deficits) in the presence of a normal brain MRI study. Focal and diffuse hypoperfusion brain lesions were found in 73% to 80% of the patients, mainly over the territory of the medial cerebral arteries. These studies demonstrated that brain SPECT is a sensitive diagnostic tool useful in identifying early neuropsychiatric involvement in patients with APS. Sun and colleagues [196] recently used brain SPECT to assess the effects of anticoagulant therapy on regional cerebral blood flow in 16 patients with primary APS and neuropsychiatric manifestations. All the patients presented with minor neuropsychiatric manifestations (headaches, cognitive dysfunction, depression) and had a normal brain MRI but abnormal findings on SPECT scan at the time of study entry. A follow-up SPECT study was repeated 1 month after anticoagulant therapy. All patients had a complete clinical recovery. Improvement in cerebral blood flow was demonstrated in all 16 patients, with a complete normalization of the hypoperfusion lesions in 70% of the cases. The authors suggested that brain SPECT is useful to assess the effects of anticoagulant therapy by determining changes on regional blood flow in APS patients with brain involvement.

Summary

The importance of cerebral disease in patients with the Hughes syndrome is now becoming more widely recognized. The range of neuropsychiatric manifestations of APS is comprehensive, and includes focal symptoms attributable to lesions in a specific area of the brain as well as diffuse or global dysfunction. Patients with APS frequently present with strokes and TIA, but a wide spectrum of other neurologic features—also including nonthrombotic neurologic syndromes—has been described in association with the presence of aPL. The recognition of APS has had a profound impact on the understanding and management of the treatment of CNS manifestations associated with connective tissue diseases, in particular, SLE. Many patients with focal neurologic manifestations and aPL, who a few years ago would have received high-dose corticosteroids or immunosuppression, are often successfully treated with anticoagulation [197]. In our opinion, testing for aPL may have a major diagnostic and therapeutic impact not only in patients with autoimmune diseases and neuropsychiatric manifestations, but also in young individuals who develop cerebral ischemia, in those with atypical multiple sclerosis, transverse myelitis, and atypical seizures. We would also recommend testing for aPL for young individuals found with multiple hyperintensity lesions on brain MRI in the absence of other possible causes, especially when under the age of 40 years. It is our practice to anticoagulate patients with aPL suffering from cerebral ischemia with a target INR of 3.0 to prevent recurrences. Low-dose aspirin alone (with occasional exceptions) does not seem helpful to prevent recurrent thrombosis in these patients. Our recommendation, once the patient has had a proven thrombosis associated with aPL, is long-term (possibly life-long) warfarin therapy [6,198]. Oral anticoagulation carries a risk of hemorrhage, but in our experience the risk of serious bleeding in patients with APS and previous thrombosis treated with oral anticoagulation to a target INR of 3.5 was similar to that in groups of patients treated with lower target ratios [199].

Although a double-blind crossover trial comparing low molecular weight heparin with placebo in patients with aPL and chronic headaches did not show a significant difference in the beneficial effect of low molecular weight heparin versus placebo [200], in our experience selected patients with aPL and neuropsychiatric manifestations such as seizures, severe cognitive dysfunction, and intractable headaches unresponsive to conventional treatment [180] may respond to anticoagulant treatment.

The neurologic ramifications of Hughes syndrome are extensive, and it behoves clinicians in all specialities to be aware of this syndrome because treatment with anticoagulation may profoundly change the outlook for these patients.

References

[1] Wilson WA, Gharavi AE, Koike T, et al. International consensus statement on preliminary classification criteria for definite antiphospholipid syndrome: report of an international workshop. Arthritis Rheum 1999;42:1309–11.

[2] Miyakis S, Lockshin MD, Atsumi T, et al. International consensus statement on an update of the classification criteria for definite antiphospholipid syndrome (APS). J Thromb Haemost 2006;4:295–306.

[3] Cervera R, Piette JC, Font J, et al. Antiphospholipid syndrome: clinical and immunologic manifestations and patterns of disease expression in a cohort of 1,000 patients. Arthritis Rheum 2002;46:1019–27.

[4] Khamashta MA, Bertolaccini ML, Hughes GR. Antiphospholipid (Hughes) syndrome. Autoimmunity 2004;37:309–12.

[5] Sanna G, Bertolaccini ML, Hughes GR. Hughes syndrome, the antiphospholipid syndrome: a new chapter in neurology. Ann N Y Acad Sci 2005;1051:465–86.

[6] Sanna G, Bertolaccini ML, Cuadrado MJ, et al. Central nervous system involvement in the antiphospholipid (Hughes) syndrome. Rheumatology (Oxford) 2003;42:200–13.

[7] Hughes GRV. Thrombosis, abortion, cerebral disease and the lupus anticoagulant. BMJ 1983;287:1088–9.

[8] Harris EN, Englert H, Derue G, et al. Antiphospholipid antibodies in acute Guillain-Barré syndrome. Lancet 1983;ii:1361–2.

[9] Hughes GRV. The Prosser-White oration 1983. Connective tissue disease and the skin. Clin Exp Dermatol 1984;9:535–44.

[10] Harris EN, Gharavi AE, Mackworth-Young CG, et al. Lupoid sclerosis: a possible pathogenetic role for antiphospholipid antibodies. Ann Rheum Dis 1985;44:281–3.

[11] Asherson R, Mercey D, Phillips G, et al. Recurrent stroke and multi-infarct dementia in systemic lupus erythematosus: association with antiphospholipid antibodies. Ann Rheum Dis 1987;46:605–11.

[12] Cuadrado MJ, Khamashta MA, Ballesteros A, et al. Can neurologic manifestations of Hughes (antiphospholipid) syndrome be distinguished from multiple sclerosis? Analysis of 27 patients and review of the literature. Medicine (Baltimore) 2000;79:57–68.

[13] Cuadrado MJ, Khamashta MA, D'Cruz D, et al. Migraine in Hughes syndrome. Heparin as a therapeutic trial? Q J Med 2001;94:114–5.

[14] Hughes GR. Migraine, memory loss, and "multiple sclerosis." Neurological features of the antiphospholipid (Hughes') syndrome. Postgrad Med J 2003;79:81–3.

[15] Shoenfeld Y, Lev S, Blatt I, et al. Features associated with epilepsy in the antiphospholipid syndrome. J Rheumatol 2004;31:1344–8.

[16] Gomez-Puerta JA, Cervera R, Calvo LM, et al. Dementia associated with the antiphospholipid syndrome: clinical and radiological characteristics of 30 patients. Rheumatology (Oxford) 2005;44:95–9.

[17] Oosting JD, Derksen RH, Blokzijl L, et al. Antiphospholipid antibody positive sera enhance endothelial cell procoagulant activity—studies in a thrombosis model. Thromb Haemost 1992;68:278–84.

[18] Simantov R, LaSala JM, Lo SK, et al. Activation of cultured vascular endothelial cells by antiphospholipid antibodies. J Clin Invest 1995;96:2211–9.

[19] Del Papa N, Guidali L, Sala A, et al. Endothelial cells as target for antiphospholipid antibodies. Human polyclonal and monoclonal anti-beta 2-glycoprotein I antibodies react in

vitro with endothelial cells through adherent beta 2-glycoprotein I and induce endothelial activation. Arthritis Rheum 1997;40:551–61.

[20] Meroni P, Tincani A, Sepp N, et al. Endothelium and the brain in CNS lupus. Lupus 2003; 12:919–28.

[21] Connor P, Hunt BJ. Cerebral haemostasis and antiphospholipid antibodies. Lupus 2003; 12:929–34.

[22] Sun KH, Liu WT, Tsai CY, et al. Inhibition of astrocyte proliferation and binding to brain tissue of anticardiolipin antibodies purified from lupus serum. Ann Rheum Dis 1992;51: 707–12.

[23] Khalili A, Cooper RC. A study of immune responses to myelin and cardiolipin in patients with systemic lupus erythematosus (SLE). Clin Exp Immunol 1991;85:365–72.

[24] Katzav A, Chapman J, Shoenfeld Y. CNS dysfunction in the antiphospholipid syndrome. Lupus 2003;12:903–7.

[25] Shoenfeld Y, Nahum A, Korczyn AD, et al. Neuronal-binding antibodies from patients with antiphospholipid syndrome induce cognitive deficits following intrathecal passive transfer. Lupus 2003;12:436–42.

[26] Blank M, Krause I, Fridkin M, et al. Bacterial induction of autoantibodies to beta2-glyco-protein-I accounts for the infectious etiology of antiphospholipid syndrome. J Clin Invest 2002;109:797–804.

[27] Shrot S, Katzav A, Korczyn AD, et al. Behavioral and cognitive deficits occur only after prolonged exposure of mice to antiphospholipid antibodies. Lupus 2002;11:736–43.

[28] Ziporen L, Polak-Charcon S, Korczyn DA, et al. Neurological dysfunction associated with antiphospholipid syndrome: histopathological brain findings of thrombotic changes in a mouse model. Clin Dev Immunol 2004;11:67–75.

[29] Krnic-Barrie S, O'Connor CR, Looney SW, et al. A retrospective review of 61 patients with antiphospholipid syndrome. Analysis of factors influencing recurrent thrombosis. Arch Intern Med 1997;157:2101–8.

[30] Shah NM, Khamashta MA, Atsumi T, et al. Outcome of patients with anticardiolipin antibodies: a 10 year follow-up of 52 patients. Lupus 1998;7:3–6.

[31] Sastre-Garriga J, Montalban X. APS and the brain. Lupus 2003;12:877–82.

[32] Hilker R, Thiel A, Geisen C, et al. Cerebral blood flow and glucose metabolism in multi-infarct-dementia related to primary antiphospholipid antibody syndrome. Lupus 2000; 9:311–6.

[33] Terashi H, Uchiyama S, Hashimoto S, et al. Clinical characteristics of stroke patients with antiphospholipid antibodies. Cerebrovasc Dis 2005;19:384–90.

[34] Asherson RA, Khamashta MA, Gil A, et al. Cerebrovascular disease and antiphospholipid antibodies in systemic lupus erythematosus, lupus-like disease, and the primary antiphospholipid syndrome. Am J Med 1989;86:391–9.

[35] Devinsky O, Petito CK, Alonso DR. Clinical and neuropathological findings in systemic lupus erythematosus: the role of vasculitis, heart emboli, and thrombotic thrombocytopenic purpura. Ann Neurol 1988;23:380–4.

[36] Ford SE, Lillicrap D, Brunet D, et al. Thrombotic endocarditis and lupus anticoagulant. A pathogenetic possibility for idiopathic "rheumatic type" valvular heart disease. Arch Pathol Lab Med 1989;113:350–3.

[37] Nesher G, Ilany J, Rosenmann D, et al. Valvular dysfunction in antiphospholipid syndrome: prevalence, clinical features, and treatment. Semin Arthritis Rheum 1997;27: 27–35.

[38] Khamashta MA, Cervera R, Asherson RA, et al. Association of antibodies against phospholipids with heart valve disease in systemic lupus erythematosus. Lancet 1990;335: 1541–4.

[39] Krause I, Lev S, Fraser A, et al. Close association between valvar heart disease and central nervous system manifestations in the antiphospholipid syndrome. Ann Rheum Dis 2005;64: 1490–3.

[40] Sanna G, Bertolaccini ML, Cuadrado MJ, et al. Neuropsychiatric manifestations in systemic lupus erythematosus: prevalence and association with antiphospholipid antibodies. J Rheumatol 2003;30:985–92.

[41] Brey RL, Hart RG, Sherman DG, et al. Antiphospholipid antibodies and cerebral ischemia in young people. Neurology 1990;40:1190–6.

[42] Levine SR, Deegan MJ, Futrell N, et al. Cerebrovascular and neurologic disease associated with antiphospholipid antibodies: 48 cases. Neurology 1990;40:1181–9.

[43] Nencini P, Baruffi MC, Abbate R, et al. Lupus anticoagulant and anticardiolipin antibodies in young adults with cerebral ischemia. Stroke 1992;23:189–93.

[44] The Antiphospholipid Antibodies in Stroke Study (APASS) Group. Anticardiolipin antibodies are an independent risk factor for first ischemic stroke. Neurology 1993;43:2069–73.

[45] Camerlingo M, Casto L, Censori B, et al. Anticardiolipin antibodies in acute non-hemorrhagic stroke seen within six hours after onset. Acta Neurol Scand 1995;92:69–71.

[46] Levine SR, Brey RL, Sawaya KL, et al. Recurrent stroke and thrombo-occlusive events in the antiphospholipid syndrome. Ann Neurol 1995;38:119–24.

[47] Tuhrim S, Rand JH, Wu XX, et al. Elevated anticardiolipin antibody titer is a stroke risk factor in a multiethnic population independent of isotype or degree of positivity. Stroke 1999;30:1561–5.

[48] Zielinska J, Ryglewicz D, Wierzchowska E, et al. Anticardiolipin antibodies are an independent risk factor for ischemic stroke. Neurol Res 1999;21:653–7.

[49] Kenet G, Sadetzki S, Murad H, et al. Factor V Leiden and antiphospholipid antibodies are significant risk factors for ischemic stroke in children. Stroke 2000;31:1283–8.

[50] Brey RL, Abbott RD, Curb JD, et al. beta(2)-Glycoprotein 1-dependent anticardiolipin antibodies and risk of ischemic stroke and myocardial infarction: the Honolulu heart program. Stroke 2001;32:1701–6.

[51] Brey RL, Stallworth CL, McGlasson DL, et al. Antiphospholipid antibodies and stroke in young women. Stroke 2002;33:2396–400.

[52] Janardhan V, Wolf PA, Kase CS, et al. Anticardiolipin antibodies and risk of ischemic stroke and transient ischemic attack: the Framingham cohort and offspring study. Stroke 2004;35:736–41.

[53] Ginsburg KS, Liang MH, Newcomer L, et al. Anticardiolipin antibodies and the risk for ischemic stroke and venous thrombosis. Ann Intern Med 1992;117:997–1002.

[54] Muir KW, Squire IB, Alwan W, et al. Anticardiolipin antibodies in an unselected stroke population. Lancet 1994;344:452–6.

[55] Montalban J, Rio J, Khamastha M, et al. Value of immunologic testing in stroke patients. A prospective multicenter study. Stroke 1994;25:2412–5.

[56] Metz LM, Edworthy S, Mydlarski R, et al. The frequency of phospholipid antibodies in an unselected stroke population. Can J Neurol Sci 1998;25:64–9.

[57] Ahmed E, Stegmayr B, Trifunovic J, et al. Anticardiolipin antibodies are not an independent risk factor for stroke: an incident case–referent study nested within the MONICA and Vasterbotten cohort project. Stroke 2000;31:1289–93.

[58] Levine SR, Salowich-Palm L, Sawaya KL, et al. IgG anticardiolipin antibody titer >40 GPL and the risk of subsequent thrombo-occlusive events and death. A prospective cohort study. Stroke 1997;28:1660–5.

[59] The Antiphospholipid Antibodies and Stroke Study Group (APASS). Anticardiolipin antibodies and the risk of recurrent thrombo-occlusive events and death. Neurology 1997;48:91–4.

[60] Levine SR, Brey RL, Tilley BC, et al. Antiphospholipid antibodies and subsequent thrombo-occlusive events in patients with ischemic stroke. JAMA 2004;291:576–84.

[61] Ruiz-Irastorza G, Khamashta MA, Hughes GR. Antiphospholipid antibodies and risk for recurrent vascular events. JAMA 2004;291:2701.

[62] Wahl D, Regnault V, de Moerloose P, et al. Antiphospholipid antibodies and risk for recurrent vascular events. JAMA 2004;291:2701–2.

[63] Cabral AR. Antiphospholipid antibodies and risk for recurrent vascular events. JAMA 2004;291:2701.

[64] Ruiz-Irastorza G, Khamashta MA. Stroke and antiphospholipid syndrome: the treatment debate. Rheumatology (Oxford) 2005;44:971–4.

[65] Galli M, Luciani D, Bertolini G, et al. Lupus anticoagulants are stronger risk factors for thrombosis than anticardiolipin antibodies in the antiphospholipid syndrome: a systematic review of the literature. Blood 2003;101:1827–32.

[66] Lanthier S, Kirkham FJ, Mitchell LG, et al. Increased anticardiolipin antibody IgG titers do not predict recurrent stroke or TIA in children. Neurology 2004;62:194–200.

[67] Hilton DA, Footitt D. Neuropathological findings in Sneddon's syndrome. Neurology 2003;60:1181–2.

[68] Sneddon IB. Cerebro-vascular lesions and livedo reticularis. Br J Dermatol 1965;77:180–5.

[69] Levine SR, Langer SL, Albers JW, et al. Sneddon's syndrome: an antiphospholipid antibody syndrome? Neurology 1988;38:798–800.

[70] Alegre VA, Winkelmann RK, Gastineau DA. Cutaneous thrombosis, cerebrovascular thrombosis, and lupus anticoagulant—the Sneddon syndrome. Report of 10 cases. Int J Dermatol 1990;29:45–9.

[71] Sinharay R. Sneddon's syndrome: additional neurological feature in antiphospholipid (Hughes') syndrome. Postgrad Med J 2003;79:550.

[72] Asherson RA, Cervera R. Unusual manifestations of the antiphospholipid syndrome. Clin Rev Allergy Immunol 2003;25:61–78.

[73] Adair JC, Digre KB, Swanda RM, et al. Sneddon's syndrome: a cause of cognitive decline in young adults. Neuropsychiatr Neuropsychol Behav Neurol 2001;14:197–204.

[74] Frances C, Piette JC. The mystery of Sneddon syndrome: relationship with antiphospholipid syndrome and systemic lupus erythematosus. J Autoimmun 2000;15:139–43.

[75] Kalashnikova LA, Nasonov EL, Kushekbaeva AE, et al. Anticardiolipin antibodies in Sneddon's syndrome. Neurology 1990;40:464–7.

[76] Toubi E, Krause I, Fraser A, et al. Livedo reticularis is a marker for predicting multi-system thrombosis in antiphospholipid syndrome. Clin Exp Rheumatol 2005;23:499–504.

[77] Briley DP, Coull BM, Goodnight SH Jr. Neurological disease associated with antiphospholipid antibodies. Ann Neurol 1989;25:221–7.

[78] Schoning M, Klein R, Krageloh-Mann I, et al. Antiphospholipid antibodies in cerebrovascular ischemia and stroke in childhood. Neuropediatrics 1994;25:8–14.

[79] Takanashi J, Sugita K, Miyazato S, et al. Antiphospholipid antibody syndrome in childhood strokes. Pediatr Neurol 1995;13:323–6.

[80] Booth F, Yanofsky R, Ross IB, et al. Primary antiphospholipid syndrome with moyamoya-like vascular changes. Pediatr Neurosurg 1999;31:45–8.

[81] Bonduel M, Sciuccati G, Hepner M, et al. Prethrombotic disorders in children with arterial ischemic stroke and sinovenous thrombosis. Arch Neurol 1999;56:967–71.

[82] Bakdash T, Cohen AR, Hempel JM, et al. Moyamoya, dystonia during hyperventilation, and antiphospholipid antibodies. Pediatr Neurol 2002;26:157–60.

[83] Yamashita Y, Kusaga A, Koga Y, et al. Noonan syndrome, moyamoya-like vascular changes, and antiphospholipid syndrome. Pediatr Neurol 2004;31:364–6.

[84] Carhuapoma JR, Mitsias P, Levine SR. Cerebral venous thrombosis and anticardiolipin antibodies. Stroke 1997;28:2363–9.

[85] Levine SR, Kieran S, Puzio K, et al. Cerebral venous thrombosis with lupus anticoagulants. Report of two cases. Stroke 1987;18:801–4.

[86] Provenzale JM, Loganbill HA. Dural sinus thrombosis and venous infarction associated with antiphospholipid antibodies: MR findings. J Comput Assist Tomogr 1994;18:719–23.

[87] Camaiti A, Del Rosso A, Checcucci D, et al. Venous dural sinus thrombosis in a middle-aged woman with anticardiolipin antibodies. Acta Neurol Belg 1995;95:92–5.

[88] Daif A, Awada A, al-Rajeh S, et al. Cerebral venous thrombosis in adults. A study of 40 cases from Saudi Arabia. Stroke 1995;26:1193–5.

[89] Boggild MD, Sedhev RV, Fraser D, et al. Cerebral venous sinus thrombosis and antiphospholipid antibodies. Postgrad Med J 1995;71:487–9.

[90] Deschiens MA, Conard J, Horellou MH, et al. Coagulation studies, factor V Leiden, and anticardiolipin antibodies in 40 cases of cerebral venous thrombosis. Stroke 1996;27:1724–30.

[91] Herranz MT, Rivier G, Khamashta MA, et al. Association between antiphospholipid antibodies and epilepsy in patients with systemic lupus erythematosus. Arthritis Rheum 1994;37:568–71.

[92] Toubi E, Khamashta MA, Panarra A, et al. Association of antiphospholipid antibodies with central nervous system disease in systemic lupus erythematosus. Am J Med 1995;99:397–401.

[93] Verrot D, San-Marco M, Dravet C, et al. Prevalence and signification of antinuclear and anticardiolipin antibodies in patients with epilepsy. Am J Med 1997;103:33–7.

[94] Shrivastava A, Dwivedi S, Aggarwal A, et al. Anti-cardiolipin and anti-beta2 glycoprotein I antibodies in Indian patients with systemic lupus erythematosus: association with the presence of seizures. Lupus 2001;10:45–50.

[95] Gibbs JW 3rd, Husain AM. Epilepsy associated with lupus anticoagulant. Seizure 2002;11:207–9.

[96] Appenzeller S, Cendes F, Costallat LT. Epileptic seizures in systemic lupus erythematosus. Neurology 2004;63:1808–12.

[97] Mackworth-Young CG, Hughes GRV. Epilepsy: an early symptom of systemic lupus erythematosus. J Neurol Neurosurg Psychiatry 1985;48:185.

[98] Inzelberg R, Korczyn AD. Lupus anticoagulant and the late onset seizures. Acta Neurol Scand 1989;79:114–8.

[99] Echaniz-Laguna A, Thiriaux A, Ruolt-Olivesi I, et al. Lupus anticoagulant induced by the combination of valproate and lamotrigine. Epilepsia 1999;40:1661–3.

[100] Peltola JT, Haapala A, Isojarvi JI, et al. Antiphospholipid and antinuclear antibodies in patients with epilepsy or new-onset seizure disorders. Am J Med 2000;109:712–7.

[101] Eriksson K, Peltola J, Keranen T, et al. High prevalence of antiphospholipid antibodies in children with epilepsy: a controlled study of 50 cases. Epilepsy Res 2001;46:129–37.

[102] Ranua J, Luoma K, Peltola J, et al. Anticardiolipin and antinuclear antibodies in epilepsy—a population-based cross-sectional study. Epilepsy Res 2004;58:13–8.

[103] Cocito L, Favale E, Reni L. Epileptic seizures in cerebral arterial occlusive disease. Stroke 1982;13:189–95.

[104] Liou HH, Wang CR, Chou HC, et al. Anticardiolipin antisera from lupus patients with seizures reduce a GABA receptor-mediated chloride current in snail neurons. Life Sci 1994;54:1119–25.

[105] Chapman J, Cohen-Armon M, Shoenfeld Y, et al. Antiphospholipid antibodies permeabilize and depolarize brain synaptoneurosomes. Lupus 1999;8:127–33.

[106] Kent M, Alvarez F, Vogt E, et al. Monoclonal antiphosphatidylserine antibodies react directly with feline and murine central nervous system. J Rheumatol 1997;24:1725–33.

[107] Kent MN, Alvarez FJ, Ng AK, et al. Ultrastructural localization of monoclonal antiphospholipid antibody binding to rat brain. Exp Neurol 2000;163:173–9.

[108] Liou HH, Wang CR, Chen CJ, et al. Elevated levels of anticardiolipin antibodies and epilepsy in lupus patients. Lupus 1996;5:307–12.

[109] Mikdashi J, Handwerger B. Predictors of neuropsychiatric damage in systemic lupus erythematosus: data from the Maryland lupus cohort. Rheumatology (Oxford) 2004;43:1555–60.

[110] Karassa FB, Ioannidis JP, Boki KA, et al. Predictors of clinical outcome and radiologic progression in patients with neuropsychiatric manifestations of systemic lupus erythematosus. Am J Med 2000;109:628–34.

[111] Lampropoulos CE, Koutroumanidis M, Reynolds PP, et al. Electroencephalography in the assessment of neuropsychiatric manifestations in antiphospholipid syndrome and systemic lupus erythematosus. Arthritis Rheum 2005;52:841–6.

[112] Cuadrado MJ, Khamashta MA, Hughes GR. Sticky blood and headache. Lupus 2001;10: 392–3.

[113] Cuadrado MJ, Sanna G. Headache and systemic lupus erythematosus. Lupus 2003;12: 943–6.

[114] Montalban J, Cervera R, Font J, et al. Lack of association between anticardiolipin antibodies and migraine in systemic lupus erythematosus. Neurology 1992;42:681–2.

[115] Tietjen GE, Day M, Norris L, et al. Role of anticardiolipin antibodies in young persons with migraine and transient focal neurologic events: a prospective study. Neurology 1998;50:1433–40.

[116] Markus HS, Hopkinson N. Migraine and headache in systemic lupus erythematosus and their relationship with antibodies against phospholipids. J Neurol 1992;239:39–42.

[117] Rozell CL, Sibbitt WL Jr, Brooks WM. Structural and neurochemical markers of brain injury in the migraine diathesis of systemic lupus erythematosus. Cephalalgia 1998;18: 209–15.

[118] Hogan MJ, Brunet DG, Ford PM, et al. Lupus anticoagulant, antiphospholipid antibodies and migraine. Can J Neurol Sci 1988;15:420–5.

[119] Iniguez C, Pascual C, Pardo A, et al. Antiphospholipid antibodies in migraine. Headache 1991;31:666–8.

[120] Hering R, Couturier EG, Steiner TJ, et al. Anticardiolipin antibodies in migraine. Cephalalgia 1991;11:19–21.

[121] Tsakiris DA, Kappos L, Reber G, et al. Lack of association between antiphospholipid antibodies and migraine. Thromb Haemost 1993;69:415–7.

[122] Robbins L. Migraine and anticardiolipin antibodies—case reports of 13 patients, and the prevalence of antiphospholipid antibodies in migraineurs. Headache 1991;31:537–9.

[123] Verrotti A, Cieri F, Pelliccia P, et al. Lack of association between antiphospholipid antibodies and migraine in children. Int J Clin Lab Res 2000;30:109–11.

[124] Asherson RA, Derksen RH, Harris EN, et al. Chorea in systemic lupus erythematosus and "lupus-like" disease: association with antiphospholipid antibodies. Semin Arthritis Rheum 1987;16:253–9.

[125] Khamashta MA, Gil A, Anciones B, et al. Chorea in systemic lupus erythematosus: association with antiphospholipid antibodies. Ann Rheum Dis 1988;47:681–3.

[126] Asherson RA, Hughes GRV. Antiphospholipid antibodies and chorea. J Rheumatol 1988; 15:377–9.

[127] Cervera R, Asherson RA, Font J, et al. Chorea in the antiphospholipid syndrome. Clinical, radiologic, and immunologic characteristics of 50 patients from our clinics and the recent literature. Medicine (Baltimore) 1997;76:203–12.

[128] Milanov IG, Rashkov R, Baleva M, et al. Antiphospholipid syndrome and parkinsonism. Clin Exp Rheumatol 1998;16:623–4.

[129] Milanov I, Bogdanova D. Antiphospholipid syndrome and dystonia-parkinsonism. A case report. Parkinsonism Relat Disord 2001;7:139–41.

[130] Reiblat T, Polishchuk I, Dorodnikov E, et al. Primary antiphospholipid antibody syndrome masquerading as progressive supranuclear palsy. Lupus 2003;12:67–9.

[131] Adhiyaman V, Meara RJ, Bhowmick BK. Antiphospholipid syndrome and dystonia-parkinsonism: need for anticoagulation. Parkinsonism Relat Disord 2002;8:215.

[132] Scott TF, Hess D, Brillman J. Antiphospholipid antibody syndrome mimicking multiple sclerosis clinically and by magnetic resonance imaging. Arch Intern Med 1994;154:917–20.

[133] Ijdo J, Conti-Kelly AM, Greco P, et al. Anti-phospholipid antibodies in patients with multiple sclerosis and MS-like illnesses: MS or APS? Lupus 1999;8:109–15.

[134] Tourbah A, Clapin A, Gout O, et al. Systemic autoimmune features and multiple sclerosis: a 5-year follow-up study. Arch Neurol 1998;55:517–21.

[135] Sastre-Garriga J, Reverter JC, Font J, et al. Anticardiolipin antibodies are not a useful screening tool in a nonselected large group of patients with multiple sclerosis. Ann Neurol 2001;49:408–11.

[136] Heinzlef O, Weill B, Johanet C, et al. Anticardiolipin antibodies in patients with multiple sclerosis do not represent a subgroup of patients according to clinical, familial, and biological characteristics. J Neurol Neurosurg Psychiatry 2002;72:647–9.

[137] Figved N, Klevan G, Myhr KM, et al. Neuropsychiatric symptoms in patients with multiple sclerosis. Acta Psychiatr Scand 2005;112:463–8.

[138] Diaz-Olavarrieta C, Cummings JL, Velazquez J, et al. Neuropsychiatric manifestations of multiple sclerosis. J Neuropsychiatr Clin Neurosci 1999;11:51–7.

[139] Nortvedt MW, Riise T, Myhr KM, et al. Quality of life as a predictor for change in disability in MS. Neurology 2000;55:51–4.

[140] Ferreira S, D'Cruz DP, Hughes GR. Multiple sclerosis, neuropsychiatric lupus and antiphospholipid syndrome: where do we stand? Rheumatology (Oxford) 2005;44:434–42.

[141] Paran D, Chapman J, Korczyn AD, et al. Evoked potential studies in the antiphospholipid syndrome: differential diagnosis from multiple sclerosis. Ann Rheum Dis 2006;65: 525–8.

[142] Kim JH, Lee SI, Park SI, et al. Recurrent transverse myelitis in primary antiphospholipid syndrome—case report and literature review. Rheumatol Int 2004;24:244–6.

[143] Alarcon-Segovia D, Deleze M, Oria CV, et al. Antiphospholipid antibodies and the antiphospholipid syndrome in systemic lupus erythematosus. A prospective analysis of 500 consecutive patients. Medicine (Baltimore) 1989;68:353–65.

[144] Lavalle C, Pizarro S, Drenkard C, et al. Transverse myelitis: a manifestation of systemic lupus erythematosus strongly associated with antiphospholipid antibodies. J Rheumatol 1990;17:34–7.

[145] Kovacs B, Lafferty TL, Brent LH, et al. Transverse myelopathy in systemic lupus erythematosus: an analysis of 14 cases and review of the literature. Ann Rheum Dis 2000;59: 120–4.

[146] D'Cruz DP, Mellor-Pita S, Joven B, et al. Transverse myelitis as the first manifestation of systemic lupus erythematosus or lupus-like disease: good functional outcome and relevance of antiphospholipid antibodies. J Rheumatol 2004;31:280–5.

[147] Falcini F, Taccetti G, Trapani S, et al. Primary antiphospholipid syndrome: a report of two pediatric cases. J Rheumatol 1991;18:1085–7.

[148] Orefice G, De Joanna G, Coppola M, et al. Benign intracranial hypertension: a non-thrombotic complication of the primary antiphospholipid syndrome? Lupus 1995;4:324–6.

[149] Sussman J, Leach M, Greaves M, et al. Potentially prothrombotic abnormalities of coagulation in benign intracranial hypertension. J Neurol Neurosurg Psychiatry 1997;62: 229–33.

[150] Leker RR, Steiner I. Anticardiolipin antibodies are frequently present in patients with idiopathic intracranial hypertension. Arch Neurol 1998;55:817–20.

[151] Kesler A, Ellis MH, Reshef T, et al. Idiopathic intracranial hypertension and anticardiolipin antibodies. J Neurol Neurosurg Psychiatry 2000;68:379–80.

[152] Hisashi K, Komune S, Taira T, et al. Anticardiolipin antibody-induced sudden profound sensorineural hearing loss. Am J Otolaryngol 1993;14:275–7.

[153] Casoli P, Tumiati B. Cogan's syndrome: a new possible complication of antiphospholipid antibodies? Clin Rheumatol 1995;14:197–8.

[154] Tumiati B, Casoli P. Sudden sensorineural hearing loss and anticardiolipin antibody. Am J Otolaryngol 1995;16:220.

[155] Toubi E, Ben-David J, Kessel A, et al. Autoimmune aberration in sudden sensorineural hearing loss: association with anti-cardiolipin antibodies. Lupus 1997;6:540–2.

[156] Naarendorp M, Spiera H. Sudden sensorineural hearing loss in patients with systemic lupus erythematosus or lupus-like syndromes and antiphospholipid antibodies. J Rheumatol 1998;25:589–92.

[157] Green L, Miller EB. Sudden sensorineural hearing loss as a first manifestation of systemic lupus erythematosus: association with anticardiolipin antibodies. Clin Rheumatol 2001;20: 220–2.

[158] Gilburd B, Stein M, Tomer Y, et al. Autoantibodies to phospholipids and brain extract in patients with the Guillain-Barre syndrome: cross-reactive or pathogenic? Autoimmunity 1993;16:23–7.

[159] Montalban J, Arboix A, Staub H, et al. Transient global amnesia and antiphospholipid syndrome. Clin Exp Rheumatol 1989;7:85–7.

[160] Brey RL, Gharavi AE, Lockshin MD. Neurologic complications of antiphospholipid antibodies. Rheum Dis Clin North Am 1993;19:833–50.

[161] Durrani OM, Gordon C, Murray PI. Primary anti-phospholipid antibody syndrome (APS): current concepts. Surv Ophthalmol 2002;47:215–38.

[162] Reino S, Munoz-Rodriguez FJ, Cervera R, et al. Optic neuropathy in the "primary" antiphospholipid syndrome: report of a case and review of the literature. Clin Rheumatol 1997; 16:629–31.

[163] Giorgi D, Gabrieli CB, Bonomo L. The clinical-ophtalmological spectrum of antiphospholipid syndrome. Ocul Immunol Inflamm 1998;6:269–73.

[164] Frohman L, Turbin R, Bielory L, et al. Autoimmune optic neuropathy with anticardiolipin antibody mimicking multiple sclerosis in a child. Am J Ophthalmol 2003;136: 358–60.

[165] Papais-Alvarenga RM, Miranda-Santos CM, Puccioni-Sohler M, et al. Optic neuromyelitis syndrome in Brazilian patients. J Neurol Neurosurg Psychiatry 2002;73: 429–35.

[166] Wiechens B, Schroder JO, Potzsch B, et al. Primary antiphospholipid antibody syndrome and retinal occlusive vasculopathy. Am J Ophthalmol 1997;123:848–50.

[167] Au A, O'Day J. Review of severe vaso-occlusive retinopathy in systemic lupus erythematosus and the antiphospholipid syndrome: associations, visual outcomes, complications and treatment. Clin Exp Ophthalmol 2004;32:87–100.

[168] Uthman I, Najjar DM, Kanj SS, et al. Anticardiolipin antibodies in acute multifocal posterior placoid pigment epitheliopathy. Ann Rheum Dis 2003;62:687–8.

[169] Ainiala H, Loukkola J, Peltola J, et al. The prevalence of neuropsychiatric syndromes in systemic lupus erythematosus. Neurology 2001;57:496–500.

[170] Brey RL, Holliday SL, Saklad AR, et al. Neuropsychiatric syndromes in lupus: prevalence using standardized definitions. Neurology 2002;58:1214–20.

[171] Loukkola J, Laine M, Ainiala H, et al. Cognitive impairment in systemic lupus erythematosus and neuropsychiatric systemic lupus erythematosus: a population-based neuropsychological study. J Clin Exp Neuropsychol 2003;25:145–51.

[172] Afeltra A, Garzia P, Mitterhofer AP, et al. Neuropsychiatric lupus syndromes: relationship with antiphospholipid antibodies. Neurology 2003;61:108–10.

[173] Hanly JG, McCurdy G, Fougere L, et al. Neuropsychiatric events in systemic lupus erythematosus: attribution and clinical significance. J Rheumatol 2004;31:2156–62.

[174] Hanly JG, Walsh NM, Fisk JD, et al. Cognitive impairment and autoantibodies in systemic lupus erythematosus. Br J Rheumatol 1993;32:291–6.

[175] Denburg SD, Carbotte RM, Ginsberg JS, et al. The relationship of antiphospholipid antibodies to cognitive function in patients with systemic lupus erythematosus. J Int Neuropsychol Soc 1997;3:377–86.

[176] Hanly JG, Hong C, Smith S, et al. A prospective analysis of cognitive function and anticardiolipin antibodies in systemic lupus erythematosus. Arthritis Rheum 1999;42(4): 728–34.

[177] Menon S, Jameson-Shortall E, Newman SP, et al. A longitudinal study of anticardiolipin antibody levels and cognitive functioning in systemic lupus erythematosus. Arthritis Rheum 1999;42:735–41.

[178] Caronti B, Calderaro C, Alessandri C, et al. Serum anti-beta2-glycoprotein I antibodies from patients with antiphospholipid antibody syndrome bind central nervous system cells. J Autoimmun 1998;11:425–9.

[179] Katzav A, Pick CG, Korczyn AD, et al. Hyperactivity in a mouse model of the antiphospholipid syndrome. Lupus 2001;10:496–9.

[180] Hughes G, Cuadrado M, Khamashta M, et al. Headache and memory loss: rapid response to heparin in the antiphospholipid syndrome. Lupus 2001;10:778.

[181] Kushner M, Simonian N. Lupus anticoagulants, anticardiolipin antibodies, and cerebral ischemia. Stroke 1989;20:225–9.

[182] Montalban J, Fernandez J, Arderiu A, et al. Multi-infarct dementia associated with antiphospholipid antibodies. Presentation of 2 cases. Med Clin (Barc) 1989;93:424–6.

[183] Kurita A, Hasunuma T, Mochio S, et al. A young case with multi-infarct dementia associated with lupus anticoagulant. Intern Med 1994;33:373–5.

[184] Mosek A, Yust I, Treves TA, et al. Dementia and antiphospholipid antibodies. Dement Geriatr Cogn Disord 2000;11:36–8.

[185] Chapman J, Abu-Katash M, Inzelberg R, et al. Prevalence and clinical features of dementia associated with the antiphospholipid syndrome and circulating anticoagulants. J Neurol Sci 2002;203–204:81–4.

[186] Schwartz M, Rochas M, Weller B, et al. High association of anticardiolipin antibodies with psychosis. J Clin Psychiatry 1998;59:20–3.

[187] Bodani M, Kopelman MD. A psychiatric perspective on the therapy of psychosis in systemic lupus erythematosus. Lupus 2003;12:947–9.

[188] Sanna G, Piga M, Terryberry JW, et al. Central nervous system involvement in systemic lupus erythematosus: cerebral imaging and serological profile in patients with and without overt neuropsychiatric manifestations. Lupus 2000;9:573–83.

[189] Vermeer SE, Den Heijer T, Koudstaal PJ, et al. Incidence and risk factors of silent brain infarcts in the population-based Rotterdam Scan Study. Stroke 2003;34:392–6.

[190] Vermeer SE, Prins ND, den Heijer T, et al. Silent brain infarcts and the risk of dementia and cognitive decline. N Engl J Med 2003;348:1215–22.

[191] Steens SC, Bosma GP, Steup-Beekman GM, et al. Association between microscopic brain damage as indicated by magnetization transfer imaging and anticardiolipin antibodies in neuropsychiatric lupus. Arthritis Res Ther 2006;8:R38.

[192] Kao CH, Lan JL, Hsieh JF, et al. Evaluation of regional cerebral blood flow with 99mTc-HMPAO in primary antiphospholipid antibody syndrome. J Nucl Med 1999; 40:1446–50.

[193] Romanowicz G, Lass P, Koseda-Dragan M, et al. Technetium-99mTc-HMPAO brain SPECT in antiphospholipid syndrome—preliminary data. Nucl Med Rev Cent East Eur 2000;3:17–20.

[194] Tokumaru S, Yoshikai T, Uchino A, et al. Technetium-99m-ECD SPECT in antiphospholipid antibody syndrome: a drastic improvement in brain perfusion by antiplatelet therapy. Eur Radiol 2001;11:2611–5.

[195] Chen JJ, Shiau YC, Wang JJ, et al. Abnormal regional cerebral blood flow in primary antiphospholipid antibody syndrome patients with normal magnetic resonance imaging findings. A preliminary report. Scand J Rheumatol 2002;31:89–93.

[196] Sun SS, Liu FY, Tsai JJ, et al. Using 99mTc HMPAO brain SPECT to evaluate the effects of anticoagulant therapy on regional cerebral blood flow in primary antiphospholipid antibody syndrome patients with brain involvement—a preliminary report. Rheumatol Int 2003;23:301–4.

[197] Sanna G, Bertolaccini ML, Mathieu A. Central nervous system lupus: a clinical approach to therapy. Lupus 2003;12:935–42.

[198] Khamashta MA, Cuadrado MJ, Mujic F, et al. The management of thrombosis in the antiphospholipid-antibody syndrome. N Engl J Med 1995;332:993–7.

[199] Ruiz-Irastorza G, Khamashta MA, Hunt BJ, et al. Bleeding and recurrent thrombosis in definite antiphospholipid syndrome: analysis of a series of 66 patients treated with oral anticoagulation to a target international normalized ratio of 3.5. Arch Intern Med 2002;162: 1164–9.

[200] Cuadrado MJ, Sanna G, Sharief M, et al. Double blind, crossover, randomised trial comparing low molecular weight heparin versus placebo in the treatment of chronic headache in patients with antiphospholipid antibodies. Arthritis Rheum 2003;48:S364 [abstract].

RHEUMATIC
DISEASE CLINICS
OF NORTH AMERICA

ELSEVIER
SAUNDERS

Rheum Dis Clin N Am
32 (2006) 491–507

Cardiac Manifestations in the Antiphospholipid Syndrome

Felicia Tenedios, MD*, Doruk Erkan, MD,
Michael D. Lockshin, MD

*Hospital for Special Surgery, Department of Rheumatology,
Weill Medical College of Cornell University,
535 East 70th Street, New York, NY 10021, USA*

The antiphospholipid syndrome (APS) is characterized by the presence of circulating antiphospholipid antibodies (aPLs) (most commonly detected by a lupus anticoagulant test, anticardiolipin antibody ELISA [aCL], and anti-β2-glycoprotein-I antibody ELISA [β2GPI]), vascular thrombosis, and/or pregnancy loss. Antiphospholipid syndrome is a systemic autoimmune disease with diverse clinical manifestations involving different organ systems. The cardiac system is one of the major target organs in APS [1].

Cardiac manifestations of the APS range from asymptomatic valve lesions to life-threatening myocardial infarction. The most common manifestations include valve abnormalities (valve thickening and vegetations), occlusive arterial disease (atherosclerosis and myocardial infarction), intracardiac emboli, ventricular dysfunction, and pulmonary hypertension (Box 1). The heterogeneity of abnormalities is linked to the varied effects that aPL induces on endothelial cells and to the different functions of endothelial cells in different anatomic sites. Autoantibody-mediated endothelial cell activation probably sustains a proadhesive, proinflammatory, and procoagulant phenotype. Furthermore, platelet activation followed by binding of aPL to platelet membrane phospholipid-bound proteins may initiate platelet adhesion and thrombosis [2]. Antiphospholipid antibodies also inhibit phospholipid-catalyzed reactions in the coagulation cascade, for instance, activation of protein C and protein S. Complement activation is necessary for induction of aPL-associated fetal loss and of thrombosis [3]. Thrombosis may represent the final common pathway of many processes, each dependent on its own particular autoantibody profile [4].

---

* Corresponding author.
  E-mail address: tenediosf@hss.edu (F. Tenedios).

0889-857X/06/$ - see front matter © 2006 Elsevier Inc. All rights reserved.
doi:10.1016/j.rdc.2006.05.008
rheumatic.theclinics.com

Box 1. Cardiac manifestations of the antiphospholipid syndrome

- Valve abnormalities
- Vegetations
- Valve thickening
- Valve dysfunction
- Thrombotic and atherosclerotic coronary occlusion
- Ventricular hypertrophy and dysfunction
- Intracardiac thrombus
- Pulmonary hypertension

Many individuals with high titer aPL do not develop clinical APS, possibly due to a pattern of antibody specificities or to the multiple ways in which aPL cause pathology [4]. Because aPL circulate for long periods before the onset of clinical disease, many investigators favor a two-hit hypothesis to explain how aPL cause injury: the presence of aPL (first hit) induces endothelial perturbation and another condition (second hit) such as pregnancy, infection, or vascular injury, triggers thrombosis. The two-hit hypothesis may explain why patients persistently positive for aPL suffer thrombosis only occasionally [5].

Valve abnormalities

Heart valve lesions (vegetation, valve thickening, and dysfunction) are frequent in patients with APS, with and without systemic lupus erythematosus (SLE) [6], and in patients with aPL alone, occurring in 6% to 83% of the examined patients [6–8]. Valve pathology may be a risk factor for epilepsy, stroke, and other central nervous system involvement, particularly with primary APS [9]. Differences in populations examined, problems of aPL test performance, and different echocardiography techniques account for the variable prevalence of valvulopathy.

Hojnik and colleagues [10] reviewed echocardiographic studies of primary APS patients; the four largest transthoracic echocardiography (TTE) studies (168 primary APS patients) reported 32% to 38% prevalence of valve lesions compared with 0% to 5% among control subjects. Lesions most frequently involved left-sided valves, mitral more commonly affected than aortic.

Several studies using Doppler echocardiography have shown a higher prevalence of valve defects in patients suffering SLE with aPL than in those without these antibodies [11–13]. Almost 89% of patients with SLE and valve disease have aPL, compared with 44% of patients without valve involvement [14]. Using transesophageal echocardiography (TEE), which is more sensitive than TTE, Turiel and colleagues [15] found valve abnormalities in 33 of 40 (82%) of primary APS patients. This study also suggested that aCL titer >40 IgG phospholipid (GPL) units is a risk factor for thromboembolism, occurring in 25% of patients. Mitral valve thickening was the most common abnormality (63%), followed by aortic valve thickening in 32%, and tricuspid valve thickening in 8%. Mitral valve thickening also correlated with aCL titer.

Some echocardiographic studies disagree whether patients with SLE are more likely than primary APS patients to have valve disease, and whether SLE patients with and without aPL differ in prevalence of valve disease. Nesher and colleagues [16], in a meta-analysis of 13 studies, found that 48% of aPL-positive SLE patients had valve lesions compared with 21% of aPL-negative SLE patients. Valve lesions were found in 36% of primary APS patients. Nihoyannopoulos and colleagues [12] demonstrated that 50% of SLE patients with aCL titer > 100 units have valve disease compared with 37% of SLE patients with aCL 9 to 100 units and 14% of SLE patients without aPL. Khamashta and colleagues [11] reported that among aPL-positive SLE patients, 16% had valve vegetations and 38% had mitral regurgitation (versus 1.2% and 12%, respectively, of aPL-negative SLE patients). In contrast, Roldan and colleagues [17] found comparable prevalences of valve abnormalities in SLE patients with (77%) and without (72%) aPL.

Arterial thromboembolism, for instance brain infarcts, is more common in patients with valve disease [18,19]. Recently, Erdogan and colleagues [20], finding cardiac abnormalities in 84% of primary APS patients and mitral regurgitation in 77.4%, reported valve lesions in all stroke patients and in most with other arterial or venous thrombosis.

Deposits of aCL immunoglobulins and complement are found in the subendothelial connective tissue of deformed valves of APS patients. The aCL isotype is mainly IgG; it appears as a continuous ribbon-like layer along the surface of the leaflets and cusps. Complement (C1q, C3c, and C4) deposits are similar in form and location, but are more granular, suggesting immune complexes. Control valves from aPL-negative patients and control tissue specimens from an APS patient do not demonstrate such staining [21].

Histopathology of valves demonstrates superficial or intravalve fibrin deposits and reorganization: vascular proliferation, fibroblast influx, fibrosis, and calcification. This results in valve thickening, fusion, and rigidity causing disrupted function. Inflammation is not a prominent feature of this valve lesion but may be present [22]. Amital and colleagues [23] suggested that deposition of aPL in heart valves initiates an inflammatory process. Support for this hypothesis came from Afek and colleagues [24], who demonstrated that markers of endothelial cell activation are upregulated in valves of APS patients while inflammatory exudate is scant.

In an effort to understand the pathogenesis of cardiac valvulitis in rheumatic diseases, Binstadt and colleagues [25] described a new animal model of spontaneous cardiac valvulitis in the K/BxN T-cell receptor (TCR) transgenic mice that develop arthritis. Inflammation of cardiac valves occurred in 35 of 36 arthritic mice. The primarily mononuclear inflammation was restricted to the left-sided cardiac valves (mitral and aortic valves), and was accompanied by valve thickening and proliferation of elastin filaments.

β2GPI is the principal target of autoantibodies in APS. Shoenfeld and colleagues [26] suggest molecular mimicry between microbial products and β2GPI as a mechanism by which pathogenic aPL may be generated in APS. Blank and colleagues [27] showed that some anti-β2GPI deposited on patients valves are able to recognize a synthetic β2GPI-related peptide (TLRVYK) that shares common sequence with different bacterial and viral antigens, raising the possibility that bacterial antigen induces a crossreacting antibody that leads to Libman-Sacks nonbacterial endocarditis.

Qaddoura and colleagues [28] published four cases of primary APS patients with valve disease. The pathologic appearance of the valves paralleled TEE: focal, symmetric, nodular abnormalities resulting from thrombi at the coapting edges of the valve leaflets or cusps. The authors concluded that this appearance is unlikely the result of vegetations from infective endocarditis, which are usually isolated lesions and asymmetric. Furthermore, the adjoining leaflet or cusp appears normal, which is seldom the case with infective endocarditis. The thrombotic nodules interfere with proper apposition and result in regurgitation, accentuated in chronic cases by underlying fibrosis.

Valve abnormalities in patients with APS are similar to those of SLE: thickening of leaflets, and irregular nodular excrescences on the closure lines or undersurfaces of the mitral and aortic valves. They can vary from minimal thickening to severe valve distortion and dysfunction requiring surgical replacement [21]. Espinola-Zavaleta and colleagues [22] performed a 1-year TEE follow-up study on 13 primary APS patients and concluded that oral anticoagulant therapy does not lead to the disappearance of vegetations. Valve lesions persisted unchanged in six patients (46%), and new lesions appeared in the remaining seven (54%). The same investigators looked at 12 primary APS patients with 5-year follow-up and again found that oral anticoagulant treatment and aspirin was ineffective in producing lesion regression [1]. Valve lesions were unchanged in three patients and, despite treatment, new valve lesions appeared in three patients. In the remaining six patients, valve lesions progressed. Myocardial infarction occurred in nine patients, six of whom had normal coronary angiography, suggesting embolism.

Turiel and colleagues [29], in a prospective study, described valve abnormalities assessed by TEE in primary APS patients over a 5-year follow-up. Of the 56 patients with elevated aPLs at baseline, 47 (84%) had repeat TEE examinations. The first TEE showed 30 (54%) patients had mitral valve thickening. Over the 5-year follow-up, cardiac involvement was unchanged in 30 subjects (64%). New cardiac abnormalities were observed in 17 (36%) patients. Anticoagulant or platelet treatment was ineffective.

Nesher and colleagues [16] reported improvement in valve thickness and hemodynamics of four APS patients treated with corticosteroid. However,

Shahian and colleagues [30] found no effect of corticosteroid treatment on chronic mitral regurgitation in one patient with primary APS, and Hojnik and colleagues [10] stated, without presenting primary data, that steroid therapy is ineffective in the treatment of valve disease. Corticosteroid therapy may accelerate healing of valve vegetations, leading to scarring and deformity of the valves [19]. It is unclear whether corticosteroids should be used for the treatment of aPL-related valve diseases.

No systematic study on immunosuppressive or anti-inflammatory treatment of aPL-related valve disease exists. In patients with SLE and recurrent systemic embolism, surgical excision of uninfected vegetations do not prevent recurrence [17]. Only rarely (4–6%) do aPL-positive patients develop valve disease severe enough to require surgical treatment [16].

Of 39 primary APS patients followed for 10 years at the Hospital for Special Surgery, 13% eventually required cardiac valve replacement and 5% were permanently incapacitated because of cardiac disease. Nine of the 22 (41%) patients with available echocardiograms, primarily TTEs, had valve thickening or vegetations; the mitral valve was affected in four patients (one had mild regurgitation), the aortic valve was involved in two patients (one had mild and one had moderate regurgitation), and both valves were involved in three patients (all three had mild aortic regurgitation, one had mild mitral regurgitation, one had moderate mitral regurgitation, and one had mild mitral stenosis) [31].

Farzaneh-Far and colleagues [32] examined the impact of aPLs on valvular, myocardial, and arterial disease in SLE. In this large echocardiographic study of 200 SLE patients, aPL was positive in 33 patients (17%). Mitral valve nodules were more common in the aPL-positive group as was the presence of moderate to severe mitral regurgitation. IgG aPL levels were higher in patients with mitral valve nodules than those without. There were no significant differences in the prevalences of aortic valve nodules or regurgitation between aPL-positive and -negative patients.

They also found that SLE patients with positive aPLs had higher levels of circulating vascular cell adhesion molecule-1 (VCAM-1) and tumor necrosis factor (TNF) receptors. The levels of TNF receptors were higher in patients with than those without mitral valve nodules. VCAM-1 is a product of activated endothelial cells, and activated monocytes are a potential source of shed TNF receptors. The authors suggest that by inducing endothelial cell activation and monocyte recruitment, aPLs may initiate an inflammatory cascade at hemodynamically vulnerable sites leading to valvular damage [33].

Intraoperative valve inspection as well as pathologic confirmation reveals tissue destruction with significant thickening and verrucous vegetations making valve repair not feasible or inappropriate. Considering the young age of aPL patients at the time of surgical intervention and the better prognosis with intensive medical treatment, a mechanical valve substitute may be advantageous over a bioprosthesis [34].

Thrombotic/atherosclerotic coronary occlusion

Premature or accelerated atherosclerosis is an important cause of morbidity and the leading cause of mortality in patients with autoimmune rheumatic diseases. Traditional risk factors for cardiovascular disease cannot fully explain the excess risk, and additional risk factors may be attributed to inflammation and autoimmunity [35]. Both preclinical (carotid plaque) and clinical (myocardial infarction) atherosclerotic disease are more prevalent in SLE patients than in the general population [36,37]. No prospective studies confirm a similar increased risk in APS. Although some suggest that aPL is an independent risk factor for accelerated atherosclerosis, in a population of SLE patients aPL was protective against atherosclerosis [4].

Recent advances underline the role of both the innate and the adaptive immune-inflammatory mechanisms in the development of atherosclerotic plaques [38] and the potential role played by pattern-recognition receptors (Toll-like receptors and scavenger receptors), cytokines (such as IL-1, IL-6, and TNFα), chemokines, pentraxines (such as CRP and PTX3) in atherogenesis [39]. Several autoantigens and their respective autoantibodies have been identified as possible factors in the development and progression of atherosclerosis, the most important being antibodies to oxidized low density lipoprotein (LDL), β2GPI, heat shock protein (HSP) 60/65 [40,41].

β2GPI is a major antigenic target for antiphospholipid antibodies. Oxidized LDL is the principal lipoprotein found in atherosclerotic lesions, and it colocalizes with β2GPI and immunoreactive CD4 lymphocytes [42]. Anti-β2GPI antibodies are more specific for thrombosis and APS than are aCL antibodies, and recent prospective studies have shown that aCL, particularly β2GPI-dependent aCL or anti- β2GPI antibodies are important predictors for arterial thrombosis (myocardial infarction and stroke) in men [40].

In some but not all studies aPLs correlate with atherosclerosis. Anti-β2GPI antibodies have a pro-atherogenic effect. Matsuura [43] showed that β2GPI in normal subjects reduces the intake of oxidized LDL by macrophages in the vessel wall, but when anti-β2GPI antibodies are present this effect is blocked. Thus, macrophage uptake of oxidized LDL is increased, leading to accelerated atherosclerosis. If macrophages are activated by the uptake of oxidized LDL, this could result in damage to endothelial cells, and subsequent promotion of thrombosis [44].

Several studies have shown that aCL crossreacts with oxidized LDL antibodies. aCL may therefore have the same pro-atherogenic effect as oxidized LDL antibodies.

Matsuura and Lopez [43] documented oxidized LDL/β2GPI complexes in patients with systemic autoimmune diseases, implicating the complexes as atherogenic autoantigens. IgG autoantibodies to oxidized LDL/β2GPI were detected in SLE and APS patients, and were strongly associated with arterial thrombosis [40].

Another potential mechanism through which antibodies found in APS could promote atherogenesis is interference with the protective effect of high-density lipoprotein (HDL) and apolipoprotein A-I (apo A-I). HDL helps to prevent the oxidation of LDL, while apo A-I stabilizes paraoxonase, an antioxidant enzyme within the HDL particle. Patients with APS have a high frequency of antibodies to HDL and apo A-I, a large percentage of which crossreact with cardiolipin [4,45].

Atherosclerosis is an important concern in primary APS because it may enhance the cardiovascular burden and contribute further to morbidity. In the Euro-Phospholipid cohort of 1000 APS patients, myocardial infarction was the presenting manifestation in 2.8% and appeared during the evolution of the disease in 5.5% of the cohort [6]. Petri [46] found that aPL is a risk factor for atherosclerosis in SLE. In the Hopkins Lupus Cohort [46] carotid plaque by ultrasonography was equally prevalent in the aPL-positive and -negative subjects, while the incidence of myocardial infarction was 3.3% in aPL-positive and 5.9% in aPL-negative SLE patients ($P = 0.06$). Although the incidence of myocardial infarction in SLE patients aged 35 to 44 years old was estimated to be 50-fold greater in the Pittsburgh Lupus Registry than in historic age-matched controls, data regarding the relation of aCL to myocardial infarction in this population are not available [36]. In our own studies, although accelerated atherosclerosis occurs in SLE, it may not be related to any autoantibody, including aPL [47].

Baron and colleagues [48] performed ankle–brachial index (ABI) tests in 43 patients with primary APS to assess the prevalence of early atherosclerosis. The ABI is a good predictor of peripheral artery disease, stroke, and cardiovascular events in middle-aged and older populations. The study showed that abnormal ABIs are more common in primary APS than in healthy subjects. Abnormal ABIs were found in 8 of 43 (19%) patients with primary APS and 2 of 49 (4%) controls ($P = 0.026$). No correlation between abnormal ABI and traditional cardiovascular risk factors or with the presence of aPL was found.

Ames and colleagues [49], among 42 patients with aPL without SLE, found that IgG aCL titer related independently to carotid intima-medial thickness (IMT), which may be a measure of diffuse atherosclerosis; although plaque, an unequivocal manifestation of atherosclerosis, was measured in this study, no mention is made of its relation to aPL. More recently, Ames and colleagues [44] suggest that premature atherosclerosis is a possibility in primary APS patients in their fourth decade of life or older.

Medina and colleagues [50] showed that primary APS patients have a high prevalence of increased carotid IMT and a decreased lumen diameter (LDD) without atherosclerotic plaques. Patients with increased IMT had more arterial events, especially stroke, than did patients with normal IMT. The study suggested that the IMT and LDD are independent of conventional risk factors, and they may be a consequence of primary APS itself. Indirect data from animal studies as well as in vitro observations support the contention that aCL may be sufficient to increase the propensity to atherosclerosis, regardless of predisposing factors.

Young patients with objectively documented peripheral vascular disease have a high prevalence of aPL. In a prospective cohort of 4081 healthy middle-aged men, Vaarala and colleagues [51] found that a high aCL level was an independent risk factor for myocardial infarction or cardiac death. The prevalence of aCL in patients presenting with myocardial infarction is between 5% and 15%; in patients younger than 45 years old, it is 21%. Hamsten and colleagues [52] and Billi and colleagues [53] found aCL to be an independent risk factor for recurrent cardiac events, among survivors of myocardial infarction [14].

In contrast, Sletnes and colleagues [54] found no association between aCL and myocardial infarction, and reported that aCL was not a risk factor for mortality or recurrent myocardial infarction in patients who survived acute myocardial infarction. Likewise, De Caterina and colleagues [55] did not detect differences in aCL levels between unselected patients with angiographic evidence of coronary artery disease and healthy controls. Thus, routine aPL screening for myocardial infarction patients is not recommended; however, testing should be considered in young patients with coronary artery disease who do not have other obvious atherosclerosis risk factors.

Anticoagulation is usually prescribed for persons who have suffered a thrombotic coronary occlusion. Elevated plasma homocysteine is known to be a risk factor for thrombosis, and elevated plasma homocysteine seems to be implicated in the thrombotic tendency of primary APS [44]. In the Hopkins Lupus Cohort [46], hydroxychloroquine had an additional protective effect, including benefit on lupus activity, hyperlipidemia, antiplatelet and "desludging" effects, and a reduction in aPL titers (this latter point is highly controversial). Hydroxychloroquine has also reduces in vivo aPL-induced thrombus formation. (If a patient has high plasma homocysteine, the addition of folate and vitamin B12 is indicated.)

Statin treatment is associated with regression of atherosclerotic lesions and with a reduction in cardiovascular complications in patients without aPL. Statins may also influence an anti-β_2GPI-induced proadhesive and proinflammatory endothelial phenotype [5]. Fluvastatin was found to blunt the thrombogenic response (thrombus size) and inflammatory response (adhesion of leucocytes) induced by high titers of aCL antibodies in an in vivo mouse model [56]. Thus, statins may be an additional tool for treatment, and are currently being tested as an adjunctive treatment. Statins may be beneficial in APS patients by: (1) theoretically replacing warfarin in preventing thrombosis recurrences without the risk of bleeding complications; (2) being an alternative treatment in patients who display thrombotic recurrences despite a correct warfarin therapy, or in those in whom warfarin is contraindicated; and (3) representing prophylactic therapy in patients with high levels of aPL but without a history of thrombosis. Unfortunately, controlled clinical studies on the use of statins in APS have not been performed [57].

Ventricular hypertrophy and dysfunction

Left ventricular (LV) hypertrophy and systolic or diastolic dysfunction may occur in association with hypertension, valve heart disease, atherosclerotic coronary artery disease, myocarditis, and SLE, especially with active disease [37]. Limited data regarding these ventricular abnormalities and no data regarding the prevalence of LV hypertrophy (not attributable to hemodynamically significant valve disease) are available in APS.

LV mass and systolic performance can be measured using echocardiographic techniques. Doppler echocardiography is required to assess diastolic function. The prevalence of systolic and diastolic dysfunction in APS has been examined in very small studies. A cross-sectional study by Tektonidou and colleagues [58] found that various echocardiographic parameters reflecting diastolic dysfunction were associated with high titers of aCL, APS, disease duration, and pulmonary hypertension. There was gradation of severity, with more severe impairment in patients with primary APS. The gradation was particularly noticeable for prolonged deceleration time, isovolumetric relaxation time, and the E/A ratio-parameters reflecting right ventricular (RV) diastolic function. In a prospective study of 18 primary APS patients without clinically evident cardiac disease Coudray and colleagues [59] showed prolonged isovolumetric relaxation time, abnormal LV early filling pattern, and decreased myocardial lengthening rate compared with age- and sex-matched healthy controls.

Hasnie and colleagues [60] showed an association between primary APS and impaired diastolic filling as evidenced by decreased peak early filling velocity (52 ± 10 cm/s in 10 primary APS patients versus 67 ± 12 cm/s in age- and sex-matched healthy controls, $P < 0.01$). Leung and colleagues [61] demonstrated an association between isolated myocardial dysfunction (global or segmental) and aPL ($P < 0.05$) in SLE patients. In this study, four of five SLE patients with isolated LV dysfunction (two patients had congestive heart failure and two were asymptomatic) had positive aPL. Tektonidou, Coudray, and Hasnie all described LV diastolic dysfunction despite the absence of systolic dysfunction or other cardiac disease, and impairment of LV diastolic function associated with abnormalities in LV relaxation and myocardial disease.

Given the small number of patients studied, the extent to which aPL independently impacts LV size and function in the absence of other confounding processes and whether such an impact is of clinical relevance remains uncertain. Myocardial thrombotic microangiopathy (thrombosis of myocardial microcirculation) occurs both in catastrophic APS and in primary APS patients who present with myocardial infarction but normal angiography [62]. Microvascular thrombosis may result in myocardial hypertrophy and dysfunction [61]. In addition, chronic pulmonary embolism can also result in RV failure.

Studying the impact of aPL antibodies in SLE patients using echocardiography, Farzaneh-Far and colleagues [32] found clinical evidence of coronary atherosclerosis and cerebrovascular disease was similar in patients with and without aPLs. LV dimensions and systolic function were also similar in aPL-positive and -negative patients.

No published study has addressed treatment of ventricular hypertrophy and dysfunction in APS. Standard pharmacologic approaches should be used, that is, treatment of hypertension and heart failure regimens demonstrated to control symptoms and prolong life.

Intracardiac thrombi

Intracardiac thrombosis is a potentially life-threatening but rare manifestation in APS. Thrombus formation can occur in all cardiac chambers, with a predilection for the right ones, and can cause pulmonary and systemic emboli. These thrombotic events may occur on native or prosthetic valves or mural endocardium. They can be induced by placing of a venous catheter [63]. Intracardiac thrombi in patients with primary APS are usually identified in the evaluation of emboli [64].

Turiel and colleagues [15], in a study of 40 primary APS patients, noted thrombus formation more frequently on the right side of the heart, contrary to valve involvement, which is mostly on the left. Recently, Erdogan and colleagues [20] found intracardiac thrombus in 5 of 31 primary APS patients; in one, it was in the left atrial appendage (LAA). The authors suggest that in search of an embolic source in primary APS patients, the LAA should be examined especially in patients with stroke. They also add that mitral regurgitation in primary APS, by impairing LAA function, might contribute to the formation of thrombus. Antibodies are thought to contribute to the formation of intracardiac thrombi, although the mechanism is unclear.

The ability of TTE to detect intracardiac thrombi is limited, for instance because of chronic obstructive lung disease or obesity. In such patients, TEE should be performed when a search for intracardiac thrombi is indicated. TEE should also be performed in APS patients with pulmonary embolism as thrombi arising from the right atrial appendage are poorly visualized on TTE.

Thrombus may be difficult to differentiate from intracardiac tumors such as myxoma; magnetic resonance imaging (MRI) may be useful in making the distinction. Tumors are hyperintense on spin echo (SE) T2-weighted images. If gadolinium is administered, tumor enhances, but thrombus does not [64]. Myxomas are usually solitary, not calcified, and attach near the fossa ovalis of the interatrial septum [65].

Intracardiac thrombi, primarily in case reports, have been treated with aggressive anticoagulation or surgical excision. Substantial data favoring either approach do not exist. Complete resolution of thrombi with anticoagulation alone is reported, but excisional biopsy is sometimes required to exclude diagnosis of cardiac myxoma and to remove thrombus. Heightened surgical risk in these patients strongly supports an initial nonsurgical approach. Following initial treatment, lifelong prophylactic anticoagulation would seem prudent given the risk of recurrence for APS patients who cease warfarin [2].

Pulmonary hypertension

Pulmonary hypertension is one of the lethal complications of APS; it can be due to chronic recurrence of embolism or in situ thrombosis. The prevalence of pulmonary hypertension in APS is between 1.8% and 3.5%. The prevalence of aPL in patients with chronic thromboembolic pulmonary hypertension (CTEPH) varies between 10% and 20%. It is likely that CTEPH after pulmonary thromboembolism develops more frequently in the presence of aPL The role of aPL in the pathophysiology of pulmonary hypertension is unclear, but explanations include a role for activated platelets; for an interaction between aPL and endothelial cells on the pulmonary vasculature, leading to vascular remodeling; or the implication of endothelin-1, a peptide that induces vasoconstriction and stimulates the proliferation of vascular muscle cells. High levels of endothelin-1 are found in both plasma and lung tissue of patients with primary pulmonary hypertension and in plasma of patients with APS with arterial thrombosis [65].

To manage pulmonary hypertension, chronic anticoagulation is needed to prevent new thromboemboli. If pulmonary hypertension is secondary to recurrent thromboembolism, the placement of an inferior vena cava filter may be recommended. Women with pulmonary hypertension need to be aware of the high risk of maternal mortality associated with pregnancy. McMillan and colleagues [66] reported three patients with two deaths, both of which developed during pregnancy and deteriorated rapidly, with mean pulmonary artery pressures of 70 and 80 mmHg before death, occurring within 48 hours of delivery.

Long-term infusion of epoprostenol (prostacyclin) may be beneficial in treating some forms of severe secondary pulmonary artery hypertension, although it has only been shown to prolong survival in primary pulmonary hypertension. One series studied a mixed population of 33 patients with pulmonary hypertension secondary to collagen vascular disease, sarcoidosis, distal thromboembolism disease, or portopulmonary hypertension [67]. Treatment with continuous epoprostenol improved hemodynamic parameters and functional capacity. Responses appeared unrelated to the underlying cause of pulmonary hypertension, suggesting that epoprostenol may favorably impact later events in the propagation and progression of the disease, including impaired endothelial production of endogenous prostacyclin in response to high intraluminal pressures.

Results are promising in studies using bosentan, a nonselective oral endothelin receptor antagonist in patients with pulmonary hypertension, but the applicability of findings are uncertain in secondary pulmonary hypertension. The mortality remains high, and in general, the outcome in patients with pulmonary hypertension and APS is usually fatal.

Cardiovascular surgery in APS patients

Patients with APS are predisposed to vascular thrombotic events, and are at additional risk for thrombosis when they undergo surgery. Patients with aPL may be prone to excessive postoperative morbidity and mortality after cardiovascular surgical procedures. In one retrospective report, 16 of 19 patients with a positive ELISA for IgG aCL suffered major postoperative complications, and 12 died of complications related to surgical interventions [68].

APS patients who present with vascular thrombosis are treated with long-term anticoagulation, which can be challenging during the surgical period. Perioperative thromboses can occur due to withdrawal of warfarin, increased hypercoagulability despite ongoing, optimal warfarin or heparin therapy, or catastrophic exacerbation of APS. In addition to thromboses, life-threatening bleeding complications can occur during the perioperative period due to excessive anticoagulation and thrombocytopenia, which is common in APS patients [69].

Monitoring anticoagulation in the patient with APS requiring cardiac surgery remains problematic. Intraoperative heparin monitoring during cardiopulmonary bypass surgery can be challenging since APS patients with lupus anticoagulants have elevated baseline activated coagulation times (ACT) or activated partial thromboplastin times (aPTT). aPL often interfere with in vitro tests of hemostasis by impeding the anchoring of coagulation proteins to phospholipid surfaces. There is no consensus as to the optimal method for assuring adequate perioperative anticoagulation in APS. Suggested methods for monitoring include: doubling of the baseline ACT level, obtaining heparin concentrations by protamine titration rather than following ACT levels, and performing heparin–ACT titration curves preoperatively to determine patient-specific target ACT levels [70].

When an APS patient undergoes a surgical procedure, serious perioperative complications (recurrent thrombosis, catastrophic exacerbation, or bleeding) may occur despite prophylaxis. Thus, perioperative strategies should be clearly identified before any surgical procedure, pharmacologic and physical antithrombosis interventions vigorously employed, periods without anticoagulation kept to an absolute minimum, and any deviation from a normal course be considered a potential disease-related event. Strategies that may guide physicians in their preoperative, intraoperative, and postoperative management of APS patients are summarized in Box 2 [69].

Summary

Experimental evidence reveals that aPL are not only markers of APS, but also may play a causative role in the development of vascular thrombosis and pregnancy morbidity. The pathogenic mechanisms of aPL seem to be heterogeneous, including endothelial cell activation, the direct inhibition

Box 2. Recommendations for perioperative medical management of patients with APS

Preoperative assessment
- Prolonged activated partial thromboplastin time or slightly prolonged prothrombin time when known to be due to APS are *not* contraindications for surgical procedures
- Platelet count >100 × 10^9/L due to APS requires no specific therapy; thrombocytopenia does not protect against thrombosis
- Surgical and interventional procedures should be the last option in the management of patients with APS

Perioperative considerations
- Minimize intravascular manipulation for access and monitoring
- Set pneumatic blood pressure cuffs to inflate infrequently to minimize stasis in the distal vascular bed
- Avoid tourniquets
- Maintain high suspicion that any deviation from a normal course may reflect arterial or venous thrombosis

Perioperative anticoagulation
- Keep periods without anticoagulation to an absolute minimum
- Employ pharmacologic and physical antithrombosis interventions vigorously and start immediately before the operation, continuing until the patient is fully ambulating
- Be aware that patients with APS can develop recurrent thrombosis despite appropriate prophylaxis
- Be aware that current conventional doses of antithrombotic regimens can result in "underanticoagulation"; patients with APS may benefit from an aggressive approach with higher than standard doses
- Manage patients with APS whose only clinical manifestation is pregnancy morbidity as if they had vascular thrombosis

Renal transplant patients
- Perioperatively, anticoagulate all APS patients (history of thrombosis) undergoing renal transplant aggressively
- Strongly consider perioperative anticoagulation in antiphospholipid antibody positive asymptomatic patients (no history of thrombosis)

From Erkan D, Leibowitz E, Berman J, Lockshin MD. Perioperative medical management of antiphospholipid syndrome: hospital for special surgery experience, review of literature, and recommendations. J Rheumatol 2002;29(4):843–9; with permission.

of the activated protein C pathway, abnormalities in platelet function, and in complement activation. aPLs induce proadhesive, proinflammatory, and procoagulant molecules that provide a persuasive explanation for induction of thrombosis in APS. Cardiac manifestations in APS include valve abnormalities (valve thickening and vegetations), occlusive arterial disease (atherosclerosis and myocardial infarction), intracardiac emboli, ventricular dysfunction, and pulmonary hypertension. aPL may be associated with accelerated atherosclerosis in APS patients. Valve disease is the most important and most common cardiac manifestation of APS [7]. The precise mechanism by which valves become deformed is not yet fully known.

References

[1] Espinola Zavaleta N, Montes RM, Soto ME, et al. Primary antiphospholipid syndrome: a 5-year transesophageal echocardiographic followup study. J Rheumatol 2004;31:2402–7.
[2] Levine JS, Branch DW, Rauch J. The antiphospholipid syndrome. N Engl J Med 2002; 346(10):752–63.
[3] Salmon JE, Girardi G. The role of complement in the antiphospholipid syndrome. Curr Dir Autoimmun 2004;7:133–48.
[4] Mackworth-Young CG. Antiphospholipid syndrome: multiple mechanisms. Clin Exp Immunol 2004;136(3):393–401.
[5] Meroni PL, Borghi MO, Raschi E, et al. Inflammatory response and the endothelium. Thromb Res 2004;114(5–6):329–34.
[6] Cervera R, Piette JC, Font J, et al. Antiphospholipid syndrome: clinical and immunologic manifestations and patterns of disease expression in a cohort of 1,000 patients. Arthritis Rheum 2002;46(4):1019–27.
[7] Lockshin M, Tenedios F, Petri M, et al. Cardiac disease in the antiphospholipid syndrome: recommendations for treatment. Committee consensus report. Lupus 2003;12(7):518–23.
[8] Tincani A, Biasini-Rebaioli C, Cattaneo R, et al. Nonorgan specific autoantibodies and heart damage. Lupus 2005;14(9):656–9.
[9] Krause I, Lev S, Fraser A, et al. Close association between valvar heart disease and central nervous system manifestations in the antiphospholipid syndrome. Ann Rheum Dis 2005; 64(10):1490–3.
[10] Hojnik M, George J, Ziporen L, et al. Heart valve involvement (Libman-Sacks endocarditis) in the antiphospholipid syndrome. Circulation 1996;93(8):1579–87.
[11] Khamashta MA, Cervera R, Asherson RA, et al. Association of antibodies against phospholipids with heart valve disease in systemic lupus erythematosus. Lancet 1990;335(8705): 1541–4.
[12] Nihoyannopoulos P, Gomez PM, Joshi J, et al. Cardiac abnormalities in systemic lupus erythematosus. Association with raised anticardiolipin antibodies. Circulation 1990;82(2): 369–75.
[13] Cervera R, Font J, Pare C, et al. Cardiac disease in systemic lupus erythematosus: prospective study of 70 patients. Ann Rheum Dis 1992;51(2):156–9.
[14] Cervera R. Coronary and valvular syndromes and antiphospholipid antibodies. Thromb Res 2004;114(5–6):501–7.
[15] Turiel M, Muzzupappa S, Gottardi B, et al. Evaluation of cardiac abnormalities and embolic sources in primary antiphospholipid syndrome by transesophageal echocardiography. Lupus 2000;9(6):406–12.
[16] Nesher G, Ilany J, Rosenmann D, et al. Valvular dysfunction in antiphospholipid syndrome: prevalence, clinical features, and treatment. Semin Arthritis Rheum 1997;27(1):27–35.

[17] Roldan CA, Shively BK, Lau CC, et al. Systemic lupus erythematosus valve disease by transesophageal echocardiography and the role of antiphospholipid antibodies. J Am Coll Cardiol 1992;20(5):1127–34.

[18] Cervera R, Khamashta MA, Font J, et al. High prevalence of significant heart valve lesions in patients with the "primary" antiphospholipid syndrome. Lupus 1991;1(1):43–7.

[19] Galve E, Ordi J, Barquinero J, et al. Valvular heart disease in the primary antiphospholipid syndrome. Ann Intern Med 1992;116(4):293–8.

[20] Erdogan D, Goren MT, Diz-Kucukkaya R, et al. Assessment of cardiac structure and left atrial appendage functions in primary antiphospholipid syndrome: a transesophageal echocardiographic study. Stroke 2005;36(3):592–6.

[21] Ziporen L, Goldberg I, Arad M, et al. Libman-Sacks endocarditis in the antiphospholipid syndrome: immunopathologic findings in deformed heart valves. Lupus 1996;5(3):196–205.

[22] Espinola-Zavaleta N, Vargas-Barron J, Colmenares-Galvis T, et al. Echocardiographic evaluation of patients with primary antiphospholipid syndrome. Am Heart J 1999;137(5):973–8.

[23] Amital H, Langevitz P, Levy Y, et al. Valvular deposition of antiphospholipid antibodies in the antiphospholipid syndrome: a clue to the origin of the disease. Clin Exp Rheumatol 1999; 17(1):99–102.

[24] Afek A, Shoenfeld Y, Manor R, et al. Increased endothelial cell expression of alpha3beta1 integrin in cardiac valvulopathy in the primary (Hughes) and secondary antiphospholipid syndrome. Lupus 1999;8(7):502–7.

[25] Binstadt BA, Nguyen LT, Huang H, et al. Spontaneous cardiac valve inflammation in the K/BxN murine arthritis model. In: European Workshop for Rheumatology Research in Crete Session III, Abstract 70, February 24, 2006.

[26] Shoenfeld Y, Blank M, Cervera R, et al. Infectious origin of the antiphospholipid syndrome. Ann Rheum Dis 2006;65(1):2–6.

[27] Blank M, Shani A, Goldberg I, et al. Libman-Sacks endocarditis associated with antiphospholipid syndrome and infection. Thromb Res 2004;114(5–6):589–92.

[28] Qaddoura F, Connolly H, Grogan M, et al. Valve morphology in antiphospholipid antibody syndrome: echocardiographic features. Echocardiography 2005;22(3):255–9.

[29] Turiel M, Sarzi-Puttini P, Peretti R, et al. Five-year follow-up by transesophageal echocardiographic studies in primary antiphospholipid syndrome. Am J Cardiol 2005;96(4):574–9.

[30] Shahian DM, Labib SB, Schneebaum AB. Etiology and management of chronic valve disease in antiphospholipid antibody syndrome and systemic lupus erythematosus. J Card Surg 1995;10(2):133–9.

[31] Erkan D, Yazici Y, Sobel R, et al. Primary antiphospholipid syndrome: functional outcome after 10 years. J Rheumatol 2000;27(12):2817–21.

[32] Farzaneh-Far A, Roman MJ, Lockshin MD, et al. Impact of antiphospholipid antibodies on cardiovascular disease in systemic lupus erythematosus. Submitted for publication.

[33] Farzaneh-Far A, Roman MJ, Lockshin MD, et al. Impact of antiphospholipid antibodies and inflammatory markers on valvular disease in systemic lupus erythematosus. Submitted for publication.

[34] Berkun Y, Elami A, Meir K, et al. Increased morbidity and mortality in patients with antiphospholipid syndrome undergoing valve replacement surgery. J Thorac Cardiovasc Surg 2004;127(2):414–20.

[35] Doria A, Sarzi-Puttini P. Heart, rheumatism and autoimmunity: an old intriguing link. Lupus 2005;14(9):643–5.

[36] Manzi S, Meilahn EN, Rairie JE, et al. Age-specific incidence rates of myocardial infarction and angina in women with systemic lupus erythematosus: comparison with the Framingham Study. Am J Epidemiol 1997;145(5):408–15.

[37] Roman MJ, Salmon JE, Sobel R, et al. Prevalence and relation to risk factors of carotid atherosclerosis and left ventricular hypertrophy in systemic lupus erythematosus and antiphospholipid antibody syndrome. Am J Cardiol 2001;87(5):663–6.

[38] Doria A, Sherer Y, Meroni PL, et al. Inflammation and accelerated atherosclerosis: basic mechanisms. Rheum Dis Clin North Am 2005;31(2):355–62.
[39] Rattazzi M, Faggin E, Bertipaglia B, et al. Innate immunity and atherogenesis. Lupus 2005; 14(9):747–51.
[40] Matsuura E, Kobayashi K, Inoue K, et al. Oxidized LDL/beta2-glycoprotein I complexes: new aspects in atherosclerosis. Lupus 2005;14(9):736–41.
[41] Mandal K, Foteinos G, Jahangiri M, et al. Role of antiheat shock protein 60 autoantibodies in atherosclerosis. Lupus 2005;14(9):742–6.
[42] George J, Harats D, Gilburd B, et al. Immunolocalization of beta2-glycoprotein I (apolipoprotein H) to human atherosclerotic plaques: potential implications for lesion progression. Circulation 1999;99(17):2227–30.
[43] Matsuura E, Lopez LR. Are oxidized LDL/beta2-glycoprotein I complexes pathogenic antigens in autoimmune-mediated atherosclerosis? Clin Dev Immunol 2004;11(2): 103–11.
[44] Ames PR, Margarita A, Sokoll KB, et al. Premature atherosclerosis in primary antiphospholipid syndrome: preliminary data. Ann Rheum Dis 2005;64(2):315–7.
[45] Delgado Alves J, Mason LJ, Ames PR, et al. Antiphospholipid antibodies are associated with enhanced oxidative stress, decreased plasma nitric oxide and paraoxonase activity in an experimental mouse model. Rheumatology (Oxford) 2005;44(10):1238–44.
[46] Petri M. Hopkins lupus cohort. 1999 update. Rheum Dis Clin North Am 2000;26(2): 199–213.
[47] Roman MJ, Shanker BA, Davis A, et al. Prevalence and correlates of accelerated atherosclerosis in systemic lupus erythematosus. N Engl J Med 2003;349(25):2399–406.
[48] Baron MA, Khamashta MA, Hughes GR, et al. Prevalence of an abnormal ankle–brachial index in patients with primary antiphospholipid syndrome: preliminary data. Ann Rheum Dis 2005;64(1):144–6.
[49] Ames PR, Margarita A, Delgado Alves J, et al. Anticardiolipin antibody titre and plasma homocysteine level independently predict intima media thickness of carotid arteries in subjects with idiopathic antiphospholipid antibodies. Lupus 2002;11(4):208–14.
[50] Medina G, Casaos D, Jara LJ, et al. Increased carotid artery intima-media thickness may be associated with stroke in primary antiphospholipid syndrome. Ann Rheum Dis 2003;62(7): 607–10.
[51] Vaarala O, Manttari M, Manninen V, et al. Anti-cardiolipin antibodies and risk of myocardial infarction in a prospective cohort of middle-aged men. Circulation 1995;91:23–7.
[52] Hamsten A, Norberg R, Bjorkholm M, et al. Antibodies to cardiolipin in young survivors of myocardial infarction: an association with recurrent cardiovascular events. Lancet 1986;1: 113–6.
[53] Bili A, Moss AJ, Francis CW, et al. Anticardiolipin antibodies and recurrent coronary events. A prospective study of 1150 patients. Circulation 2000;102:1258–63.
[54] Sletnes KE, Smith P, Abdelnoor M, et al. Antiphospholipid antibodies after myocardial infarction and their relation to mortality, reinfarction, and non-haemorrhagic stroke. Lancet 1992;339(8791):451–3.
[55] De Caterina R, d'Ascanio A, Mazzone A, et al. Prevalence of anticardiolipin antibodies in coronary artery disease. Am J Cardiol 1990;65(13):922–3.
[56] Ferrara DE, Liu X, Espinola RG, et al. Inhibition of the thrombogenic and inflammatory properties of antiphospholipid antibodies by fluvastatin in an in vivo animal model. Arthritis Rheum 2003;48(11):3272–9.
[57] Riboldi P, Gerosa M, Meroni PL. Statins and autoimmune diseases. Lupus 2005;14(9): 765–8.
[58] Tektonidou MG, Ioannidis JP, Moyssakis I, et al. Right ventricular diastolic dysfunction in patients with anticardiolipin antibodies and antiphospholipid syndrome. Ann Rheum Dis 2001;60(1):43–8.

[59] Coudray N, de Zuttere D, Bletry O, et al. M mode and Doppler echocardiographic assessment of left ventricular diastolic function in primary antiphospholipid syndrome. Br Heart J 1995;74(5):531–5.

[60] Hasnie AM, Stoddard MF, Gleason CB, et al. Diastolic dysfunction is a feature of the antiphospholipid syndrome. Am Heart J 1995;129(5):1009–13.

[61] Leung WH, Wong KL, Lau CP, et al. Association between antiphospholipid antibodies and cardiac abnormalities in patients with systemic lupus erythematosus. Am J Med 1990;89(4): 411–9.

[62] Asherson RA, Cervera R, Piette JC, et al. Catastrophic antiphospholipid syndrome. Clinical and laboratory features of 50 patients. Medicine (Baltimore) 1998;77(3):195–207.

[63] Granel B, Garcia E, Serratrice J, et al. Asymptomatic intracardiac thrombi and primary antiphospholipid syndrome. Cardiology 1999;92(1):65–7.

[64] Erkan D, Erel H, Yazici Y, et al. The role of cardiac magnetic resonance imaging in antiphospholipid syndrome. J Rheumatol 2002;29(12):2658–9.

[65] Espinosa G, Cervera R, Font J, et al. The lung in the antiphospholipid syndrome. Ann Rheum Dis 2002;61(3):195–8.

[66] McMillan E, Martin WL, Waugh J, et al. Management of pregnancy in women with pulmonary hypertension secondary to SLE and anti-phospholipid syndrome. Lupus 2002;11(6): 392–8.

[67] McLaughlin VV, Genthner DE, Panella MM, et al. Compassionate use of continuous prostacyclin in the management of secondary pulmonary hypertension: a case series. Ann Intern Med 1999;130(9):740–3.

[68] Ciocca RG, Choi J, Graham AM. Antiphospholipid antibodies lead to increased risk in cardiovascular surgery. Am J Surg 1995;170(2):198–200.

[69] Erkan D, Leibowitz E, Berman J, et al. Perioperative medical management of antiphospholipid syndrome: hospital for special surgery experience, review of literature, and recommendations. J Rheumatol 2002;29(4):843–9.

[70] East CJ, Clements F, Mathew J, et al. Antiphospholipid syndrome and cardiac surgery: management of anticoagulation in two patients. Anesth Analg 2000;90(5):1098–101.

ELSEVIER
SAUNDERS

Rheum Dis Clin N Am
32 (2006) 509–522

RHEUMATIC
DISEASE CLINICS
OF NORTH AMERICA

Kidney Disease in Antiphospholipid Syndrome

Mary-Carmen Amigo, MD, FACP

*Universidad Nacional Autónoma de México, Department of Rheumatology,
Instituto Nacional de Cardiología Ignacio Chávez, Juan Badiano #1,
Distrito Federal, Tlalpan, Mexico 14080, Mexico*

The kidney is a major target organ in patients with the antiphospholipid syndrome (APS). However, it is only in the past few years that knowledge about renal vascular involvement in APS has acquired a critical mass. This can be explained because APS was first described in patients with systemic lupus erythematosus (SLE) and the studies were focused on the immune complex-mediated glomerulonephritis rather than the renal vascular lesions. In addition, the risks of a renal biopsy in APS patients because of the frequent occurrence of thrombocytopenia and systemic hypertension, discouraged the procedure and impeded the pathologic demonstration of intrarenal thrombotic lesions.

The renal manifestations may result from thrombosis occurring at any location within the renal vasculature, including large vessels, both arterial and venous, the intraparenchymatous arteries and arterioles, as well as the glomerular capillaries. However, other types of renal involvement including membranous glomerulonephritis, pauci-immune crescentic glomerulonephritis, IgA nephropathy, focal segmental glomerulosclerosis, glomerulonephritis with isolated C3 mesangial deposits, and vasculitis associated with aPL have all been described. It is unclear whether, in addition to thrombosis, other mechanisms could also contribute to the pathogenesis of the nephropathy of APS (NAPS). The consequences of the renal compromise include renovascular hypertension, renal infarcts, cortical atrophy, acute renal failure, proteinuria, and end stage renal disease (Table 1).

There is a prevailing opinion that given its importance and unique features, the NAPS, should be included in the APS classification criteria. In this review, I will discuss systemic hypertension, renal artery lesions, the

E-mail address: marycarmenamigo@gmail.com (M-C. Amigo).

doi:10.1016/j.rdc.2006.05.004

rheumatic.theclinics.com

Table 1
Kidney vascular involvement in APS

Vascular lesion	Clinical consequences
Renal artery lesions	Renovascular hypertension (severe)
Thrombosis/occlusion/stenosis?	Renal infarcts (silent, painful, hematuria)
Glomerular capillary thrombosis	Increased likelihood of renal insufficiency
leading to glomerular sclerosis	
(studied mainly in SLE)	
Renal thrombotic microangiopathy	Systemic hypertension (usually severe)
-Glomerular capillaries	Renal failure
-Arteriolar fibrous occlusions	Proteinuria (mild to nephrotic range)
-Fibrous intima hyperplasia of interlobular	Hematuria
arteries and their branches with/without	
focal or difusse cortical necrosis	
-Cortical atrophy	
Renal vein thrombosis	Risk of renal failure (if bilateral)

Abbreviations: APS, antiphospholipid syndrome; SLE, systemic lupus erythemaosus.

Adapted from Amigo MC and García-Torres R. Kidney disease in antiphospholipid syndrome. In: Khamashta MA, Editor. Hughes Syndrome Antiphospholipid Syndrome. Springer-Verlag, London; 2000. p. 70–81.

NAPS, renal vein thrombosis, the significance of antiphospholipid antibodies (aPL) in patients with SLE, and the relevance of aPL in end stage renal failure and renal transplantation.

Systemic hypertension

Hypertension (HT) is a common feature of the APS both in the primary and the secondary forms [1–4]. It appears to be a marker of nephropathy as it has been consistently present in the majority of patients with APS and renal involvement. It is important to keep in mind that both microvasculopathy or occlusion of the renal artery can contribute to severe HT in APS [1,5]. The prevalence of HT in 600 patients with primary APS (n = 68), secondary APS (n = 522), or positive for aPL (n = 10) at St Thomas' Lupus Clinic was 29%, and it was associated with livedo reticularis in 86% of the cases [6]. In primary APS, in our series of five patients with thrombotic microangiopathy [1], severe hypertension was present in all five patients and in the series by Nochy and colleagues [4], HT was present in 93% of their 16 patients with intrarenal vascular lesions. Malignant hypertension in APS without overt lupus nephritis or stenosis/thrombosis of the main renal arteries was documented by Cacoub and colleagues in five patients. Interestingly, high-dose steroids and anticoagulation led to rapid resolution of the hypertensive crisis in three of their patients [2].

The pathophysiology of HT in the context of primary APS includes thrombosis/occlusion of the trunk of a renal artery leading to renovascular hypertension as well as stimulation of the renin–angiotensin–aldosterone system secondary to intrarenal vascular lesions. Once HT is established, it may worsen vascular lesions [4]. Clinicians should thus investigate HT in all APS patients and treat them accordingly.

Renal artery lesions

Renal artery occlusion/stenosis has been reported in patients with aPL, both in the context of rheumatic conditions, mainly SLE, or in the primary APS. Early reports described unilateral or bilateral renal artery stenosis (RAS) or thrombosis with renal cortical ischemia or renal infarction [7–10]. Of particular interest are the communications by Rossi and colleagues [11] and Mandreoli and colleagues [12,13] regarding cases of renovascular HT with renal artery stenosis, which suggested a pathogenetic link between renal artery stenosis, thrombosis, fibromuscular dysplasia (FD) and aPL. Recently, a significantly increased prevalence of RAS (26%) was found in 20 out of 77 patients with aPL and hypertension (60 with SLE + APS, 11 with primary APS, and 6 with aPL only), compared with 8% of 91 relatively young hypertensive controls and 3% in 92 healthy potential renal donors [5]. In this study, magnetic resonance imaging angiography (MRA) was used to image the renal arteries. In sixteen of the patients, a smooth, well-delineated stenosis was present in the proximal third of the artery. The remaining four patients had irregular, tortuous renal arteries and aorta, suggesting atherosclerotic lesions. Three of the patients had irregular renal arteries without evidence of stenosis. In five young hypertensive patients the appearance was suggestive of fibromuscular dysplasia. MRA was repeated in five patients for suspected restenosis of the angioplasty/stents, which was documented in two. One of these patients was not anticoagulated and the other had a low international normalized ratio (<2.3).

The smooth stenotic lesions in the midportion of the renal artery are quite different from either FD or atherosclerosis (AT). FD is a hyperplastic disorder affecting medium size and small arteries. The histologic classification of FD includes intimal, medial, and periadventitial dysplasia. Medial dysplasia is the most common type and is characterized by hyperplasia of the media with or without fibrosis of the elastic membrane. It is identified angiographically by a "string of beads" appearance caused by thickened fibromuscular ridges contiguous with thin, less involved portions of the arterial wall [14]. On the other hand, in AT the atheromatous plaque is located at the origin of the renal artery and is characteristic of older patients [14].

Even though the nature of the renal artery stenosis in APS remains unclear, the response to anticoagulation does suggest a thrombotic process. However, accelerated atherosclerosis as well as increased endothelin levels with subsequent vasoconstriction have also been considered as etiologic factors [5]. It cannot be overemphasized that in cases of RAS of unknown origin, APS must be excluded.

Successful treatment with antihypertensive drugs [11,15], aspirin [16], anticoagulant therapy [10,12], and transluminal angioplasty with or without stenting has been reported [9,17,18]. Surgery, however, is restricted to those patients in whom angioplasty and stenting are not feasible. It is crucial to remember that the sooner an arterial lesion is relieved, the likelier a successful outcome.

Intrarenal vascular lesions—The nephropathy of antiphospholipid syndrome

The most commonly reported intrarenal vascular lesion in patients with aPL is thrombotic microangiopathy (TMA) (Figs. 1–3). This condition was initially described in patients with SLE [19–21] and in patients with lupus anticoagulant (LA) and pregnancy-related renal failure [22]. Subsequently, isolated cases of TMA in patients with primary APS were reported [23,24]. In our original series, published in 1992, we described five patients who had renal disease and HT among 20 consecutive patients with primary APS [1]. Mild renal failure was present in three patients while two had end-stage renal disease requiring hemodyalisis. In addition, proteinuria from mild to nephrotic was also present. The study of the kidney biopsies allowed us to observe the lesions due to APS in its pure form. Biopsy findings in all five patients were consistent with TMA. Microangiopathy involved both the vascular tree and the glomerular tufts with acute as well as old and recanalizing thrombi. Subsequently, these findings have consistently been found in the literature. Nochy and colleagues [4] in a retrospective study of 16 patients with primary APS confirmed our initial observations on glomerular and interlobular arteriolar lesions (Figs. 4 and 5). In addition,

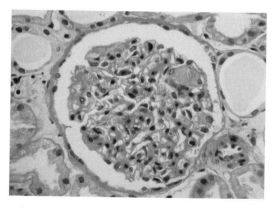

Fig. 1. Renal biopsy from an APS patient showing one glomerulus with retraction of the glomerular tuft and wrinkling of the glomerular basement membranes of the capillary wall. The presence of thrombi is also evident (PAS 400×). (Courtesy of M.C. Avila, MD, Mexico City, Mexico.)

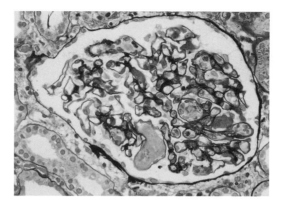

Fig. 2. Renal section showing one glomerulus increased in size that presents micro thrombi. The early presence of double contours and cellular interposition is appreciated by the Jones's stain (Jones stain 400×). (Courtesy of M.C. Avila, MD, Mexico City, Mexico.)

they emphasized the presence of focal cortical atrophy (FCA) involving the superficial cortex under the renal capsule, as foci or triangles leading to tissue retraction. These authors considered the NAPS as an entity in its own right being characterized by TMA, fibrous intimal hyperplasia (FIH) of the arteries and arterioles, and FCA. Moreover, some glomerular ultraestructural changes have recently been proposed as pathognomonic of NAPS [25], namely glomerular basement membrane wrinkling and reduplication. On electron microscopy, redundant wrinkled segments of basement membrane with straighter thin basement membrane adjacent to the endothelium are shown. However, these findings must await confirmation in larger studies.

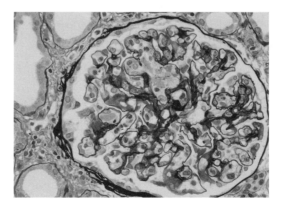

Fig. 3. Glomerular thrombotic microangiopathy. Double contours and cellular interposition are seen (Jones stain 400×). (Courtesy of M.C. Avila, MD, Mexico City, Mexico.)

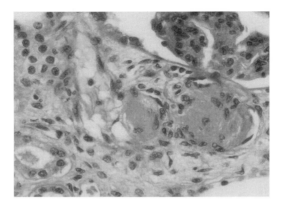

Fig. 4. Cross-section of a small artery occluded by fibrin-like material. Hematoxylin and eosin, ×400. (Courtesy of Beatriz De Leon, MD.)

It is worth mentioning that TMA is not exclusive for APS, but occurs in many other entities caused by coagulation disturbances or endothelial cell injury, which result in the formation of thrombi within the renal vasculature. These conditions include thrombotic thrombocytopenic purpura (TTP), hemolytic uraemic syndrome (HUS), scleroderma renal crisis, malignant hypertension, pre-eclampsia, and postpartum renal failure. Contraceptives, cyclosporine toxicity, chemotherapy, and renal transplant rejection are additional etiologic factors [26].

It can be very difficult to differentiate between APS, particularly the catastrophic APS (CAPS), SLE, and the TTP/HUS coagulopathies. They not only share TMA, but central nervous system symptoms, thrombocytopenia, and hemolysis. Moreover, they can occur simultaneously. Not surprisingly, APS and the HUS/TTP share endothelial injury and thrombus formation as

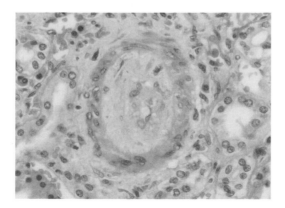

Fig. 5. Small interlobular artery with considerable intimal thickening. Hematoxylin and eosin, ×400. (Courtesy of Beatriz De Leon, MD.)

pathogenic mechanisms. In the CAPS, severe multiorgan dysfunction secondary to small vessel thrombosis and ischaemia dominates the clinical picture. Severe hypertension due to renal artery/vein thrombosis or thrombotic microangiopathy is common in CAPS patients [27].

Recently, there have been reports of histologic documentation of other types of renal involvement in patients with primary APS. These have included membranous glomerulonephritis, IgA nephropathy, pauci-immune crescentic glomerulonephritis, glomerulonephritis with isolated C3 mesangial deposits, vasculitis, and focal segmental glomerulosclerosis (FSG) [28–30]. In a retrospective study, 5 out of 270 consecutive renal biopsies were identified as biopsies performed in patients with primary APS [31]. Histologic examination of these biopsies showed tubulointerstitial lesions in all, vascular lesions and FSG in four. It is not surprising, as FSG may be a sequela of TMA. It is unclear, however, whether in addition to thrombosis, other mechanisms could also contribute to the pathogenesis of NAPS. There is evidence that anticardiolipin antibodies (aCL) recognize β-2 glycoprotein I (β2GP1) on endothelial cells leading to increased expression of adhesion molecules, increased adhesion of monocytes to endothelial cells, and complement activation [32]. These events could explain the inflammation found in the glomeruli in these uncommon cases. These findings have more than an academic interest. The distinction between renal inflammation whether caused by immune complex deposition or other causes, and microvascular thrombosis could give clues about the pathogenesis of APS and could help determine an appropriate treatment for these patients. Renal inflammation may require steroids and cytotoxic therapy, whereas APS vasculopathy benfits from anticoagulation.

The management of renal involvement in primary APS has been empirical. Hamidou and colleagues [33] reported disappearance of proteinuria and normalization of renal function with the use of aspirin and captopril in one patient with TMA and primary APS. Olguín and colleagues [34] documented renal function improvement in all five patients with NAPS with the combination of oral anticoagulants, aspirin, and nifedipine. Korkmaz and colleagues [35] found a beneficial effect of immunosuppressive therapy (azathioprine or cyclophosphamide) along with warfarin and an angiotensin-converting enzyme inhibitor in four cases with NAPS. Recently, Bhowmik and colleagues [36] reported a patient with primary APS, steroid-responsive FSG, and a successful pregnancy. However, further studies are needed to unravel the basic mechanisms of renal involvement in APS so that a targeted, more appropriate treatment be designed.

Renal vein thrombosis

Thrombosis of one or both main renal veins occurs in a variety of settings including trauma, extrinsic compression, renal cell carcinoma, nephrotic syndrome, pregnancy, and oral contraceptives. Renal vein thrombosis

(RVT) has been described in aPL positive patients with SLE [37], in a fatal case of renal transplant [38], and in patients with primary APS including a patient with bilateral RVT in the postpartum period [39,40]. Asherson [41] was the first to describe the association between aPL and RVT in two patients with SLE, proliferative nephritis and nephrotic syndrome. The clinical manifestations of RVT depend on the extent of the lesion. Acute or subacute deterioration of renal function or exacerbation of proteinuria and hematuria should alert the clinician. Even though the definitive diagnosis can only be established through selective renal venography, Doppler ultrasound, contrast-enhanced computed tomography, and magnetic resonance imaging often provides the diagnosis. Management consists of anticoagulation.

The significance of antiphospholipid antibodies in patients with systemic lupus erythematosus nephropathy

The prevalence and significance of glomerular capillary thrombosis in patients with SLE have been studied by Kant and colleagues [42] and Glueck and colleagues [37]. These authors found capillary thrombosis in near 50% of the cases with proliferative glomerulonephritis including 78% in patients with LA and 38% in those without. Notably, the presence of glomerular thrombi in the initial biopsy was a strong predictor of glomerular sclerosis. Other studies have not shown an association between aPL and prognosis in lupus nephritis. However, Moroni and colleagues [43], recently documented the impact of aPL in 111 patients with lupus nephritis followed for a mean of 173 ± 100 months. Interestingly, a strong association between aPL and the development of chronic renal failure in the long term was found. In the mutlivariate analysis, aPL positivity, high plasma creatinine level at presentation, and chronicity index, were independent predictors of chronic renal function deterioration. Miranda and colleagues [44] found no association between the presence of glomerular thrombi and severity of lupus nephritis in their analysis of 108 cases. Curiously, only nine of their patients were positive for aPL. Daugas and colleagues [3] addressed the presence and clinical relevance of NAPS in patients with SLE. This study, which was retrospective, included 114 patients with SLE nephropathy. The study showed that NAPS was present in 32% of the patients, in addition to, and independently from, lupus nephritis. NAPS was statistically associated with the presence of LA but not with anticardiolipin antibodies, and was associated with extrarenal APS, mainly arterial thrombosis and fetal loss. Finally, these authors found that NAPS is an independent risk factor contributing to hypertension, elevated serum creatinine and interstitial fibrosis. Recently, Tektonidou and colleagues [45] examined the prevalence and long-term outcome of NAPS in 151 SLE patients with or without aPL as well as the histologic evolution of NAPS lesions on serial kidney biopsies. NAPS was documented independently of lupus nephritis in two thirds of SLE patients with secondary APS, one third of SLE patients with aPL, and in only

3 out of 70 SLE patients without aPL. Progression of the acute thrombotic lesions to chronic proliferative, obstructive, and fibrotic forms was observed. TMA in the first biopsy was usually followed by chronic lesions. In addition, a strong association between NAPS, arterial thrombosis, and livedo reticularis was found in this series. All of these findings strongly suggest that patients with lupus nephritis who develop an additional NAPS should be considered for long-term anticoagulation in addition to immunosupression. Long-term prospective studies to accurately define the impact of NAPS and the role of anticoagulant or vasoprotective treatments are urgently needed.

End-stage renal disease

Patients with end-stage renal disease (ESRD) have a higher frequency of aPL positivity compared with the general population [46–49]. The prevalence of aPL is higher in hemodialysis patients compared with those on continous ambulatory peritoneal dialysis [48,49]. Quereda and colleagues [46] were the first to report the presence of LA in hemodialysis patients. The same group, in a prospective study of 138 patients with nephropathy, found that aPL was present 34% of patients with SLE, 9% in patients with chronic primary glomerulonephritis, 2.6%in patients with nonimmunologically mediated renal diseases (2.6%) [50]. Why aPL appear in hemodialysis patients is unclear. Several mechanisms have been considered including autoimmunity from an altered immune function due to uremia [51], dialysis membranes incompatibility [49], trauma to blood passing through the hemodialysis circuit [52], as well as induction by microbial agents [53]. The aPL produced in ESRD patients appear to be β2GP1-independent [54]. However, their significance remains to be clarified because, although some studies suggest that they are not pathogenic [55–58], others indicate that aPL are associated with hemodialysis vascular access thrombosis [1,59–62]. Recently, a case of CAPS following initiation of hemodialysis after bilateral nephrectomy due to renal cancer was documented. Endothelial cell damage due to arteriovenous fistula creation/cannulation, in addition to infection, and warfarin withdrawal were considered the trigger factors for the development of CAPS in this patient [63].

Renal transplantation

Reports of aPL-related morbidity among SLE kidney transplant patients are limited by the relative small number of subjects available for study at any given center. In the University of California, San Francisco study [64], a total of 97 SLE patients who underwent renal transplantation were compared with matched controls. Patients with SLE had poorer transplantation outcomes, with more than twice the risk of allograft loss. In this study, 15.4% of allograft failures were attributed to aPL-associated events. In a retrospective study of 13 SLE patients who received renal transplant,

Radakrishna and colleagues [65], compared eight patients with aCL to five patients without, transplanted during the same period. Thrombotic episodes occurred in three patients in the aCL-positive group but none in the aCL-negative group. There were no differences in the number of rejection episodes, rate of graft loss, or renal function at follow-up. These authors concluded that patients with SLE and aCL can be successfully transplanted. However, in a retrospective study of 96 consecutive patients with SLE who underwent renal transplantation, Stone and colleagues [66] assesses the impact of aPL on renal transplantation. Twenty five patients had at least one aPL. Among these 25 patients, 15 (60%) had clinical events associated with APS including 10 cases of posttransplantation morbidity or mortality attributable to the APS (three deaths, five graft losses, and two TMA).

In 1994, we reported two primary APS patients with ESRD due to TMA who underwent renal transplantation [67]. Despite intensive anticoagulant therapy, massive thrombosis of the graft in one case and TMA in the other, suggested recurrence of disease. Furthermore, our two patients had vascular access thrombosis and one had previous peritoneal dyalisis catheter malfunction due to fibrin-related obstruction. As far as we know, this was the first report of kidney transplantation in patients with primary APS.

Subsequently, there has been increasing evidence that aPL positive patients undergoing renal transplantation are at a significantly increased risk of renal vascular thrombosis, graft loss, and systemic thrombosis.

It has been demonstrated that patients with APS are at a greater risk for the development of renal allograft thrombosis within 1 week after transplantation. In a striking study, within a group of 78 patients who received renal transplant, 6 had APS. Each of these six patients thrombosed their renal allograft within a week of the transplant. In contrast, the remaining 72 patients were all doing well 1 year after transplantation [68]. In a multicenter study of 502 ESRD patients awaiting renal transplantation the potential risks associated with APS were assessed and strategies for therapeutic intervention were reviewed [69]. Twenty-three patients were diagnosed with APS. Of these, 11 received a kidney transplant either with (four patients) or without (seven patients) concomitant anticoagulation. All seven patients without anticoagulation lost their allograft within 1 week as a result of renal thrombosis. In contrast, three of the four patients who were anticoagulated maintained their allografts for over 2 years; the fourth patient lost his allograft due to thrombosis. Of the remaining 70 patients with aCL without thrombosis, 37 were successfully transplanted. Recently, the same group of investigators reported their experience with nine APS renal transplant patients [70]. Seven were treated with coumadin whereas two received heparin. Of the two patients treated with heparin, one had an early allograft loss and the other is doing well at 5 years posttransplant. Of the seven patients treated with coumadin, two are doing well, two had early allograft loss, and the remaining three returned to dialysis after they were taken off coumadin because of bleeding complications.

In another setting, it has been suggested that aPL may be implicated in the pathogenesis of TMA/HUS in a subset of hepatitis C-positive (HCV) renal allograft recipients [71]. Five HCV-positive renal transplant recipients developed biopsy-proven de novo TMA shortly after renal transplantation. Anticardiolipin antibodies were detected in pretransplant sera of these five patients and in only 1 of 13 HCV-positive recipients without TMA. In addition to TMA, three patients also presented other thrombotic complications and four of the five patients died within 5 years after transplantation. It is interesting to note that HCV infection has been associated with the development of several autoantibodies including aPL.

It has been suggested that patients with ESRD of any cause should be screened for aPL, and if detected, prevention with perioperative heparin and maintenance warfarin should be considered despite the high rate of bleeding complications, in view of the serious risk of thrombosis of the graft. Finally, in patients with APS, one should question which patients should be transplanted and which therapeutic interventions should be used because there is a high risk of posttransplant renal thrombosis even with anticoagulation. A prospective randomized multicenter study addressing these issue is warranted.

Several questions should be answered in the near future regarding the nephropathy of APS:

1. When a renal biopsy should be performed in patients with APS?
2. Are APS patients at an increased risk of bleeding during kidney biopsy?
3. What is the physiopathology of renovascular hypertension in APS?
4. What is the optimal treatment for the renal manifestations of APS?
5. What is the optimal management for APS patients undergoing kidney transplantation?

Summary

Renal involvement is a frequent finding in patients with APS. All vascular structures of the kidney may be affected, leading to diverse clinical consequences including severe hypertension, proteinuria, hematuria, nephrotic syndrome, and renal failure. In some instances ESRD may occur. Unfortunately, APS patients are at high risk of posttransplant renal thrombosis. The nephropathy of APS is characterized by TMA, FIH, and FCA. The nephropathy of APS should be included in the APS classification criteria. Prospective studies to evaluate management of the diverse renal compromise in APS patients are urgently needed.

References

[1] Amigo MC, García-Torres R, Robles M, et al. Renal involvement in primary antiphospholipid syndrome. J Rheumatol 1992;19:1181–5.
[2] Cacoub P, Wechler B, Piette JC, et al. Malignant hypertension in antiphospholipid syndrome without overt lupus nephritis. Clin Exp Rheumatol 1993;11:479–85.

[3] Daugas E, Nochy D, Huong du LT, et al. Antiphospholipid syndrome nephropathy in systemic lupus erythematosus. J Am Soc Nephrol 2002;13:42–52.

[4] Nochy D, Daugas E, Droz D, et al. The intrarenal vascular lesions associated with primary antiphospholipid syndrome. J Am Soc Nephrol 1999;10:507–18.

[5] Sangle SR, D'Cruz DP, Jan W, et al. Renal artery stenosis in the antiphospholipid (Hughes) syndrome and hypertension. Ann Rheum Dis 2003;62:999–1002.

[6] Sangle S, D'Cruz D, Khamashta M, et al. Prevalence of hypertension in 600 patients with antiphospholipid syndrome. Rheumatology (Oxford) 2004;43(suppl 2):105.

[7] Ostuni PA, Lazzarin P, Pengo V, et al. Renal artey thrombosis and hypertension in a 13 year-old girl with antiphospholipid syndrome. Ann Rheum Dis 1990;49:184–7.

[8] Hernández D, Domínguez ML, Díaz F, et al. Renal infarction in a severely hypertensive patient with lupus erythematosus and antiphospholipid antibodies. Nephron 1996;72:298–301.

[9] Asherson RA, Noble GE, Hughes GRV. Hypertension, renal artery stenosis and "primary" antiphospholipid syndrome. J Rheumatol 1991;18:1413–5.

[10] Ames PRJ, Cianciaruso B, Vellizzi V, et al. Bilateral renal artery occlusion in a patient with primary antiphospholipid antibody syndrome: thrombosis, vasculitis or both? J Rheumatol 1992;19:1802–6.

[11] Rossi E, Sani C, Zini M, et al. Anticardiolipin antibodies and renovascular hypertension. Ann Rheum Dis 1992;51:1180–1.

[12] Mandreoli M, Zuccala A, Zucchelli P. Fibromuscular dysplasia of the renal arteries associated with antiphospholipid auotantibodies: two case reports. Am J Kidney Dis 1992;20:500–3.

[13] Mandreoli M, Zucchelli P. Renal vascular disease in patients with primary antiphospholipid antibodies. Nephrol Dial Transplant 1993;8:1277–80.

[14] Safian RD, Textor SC. Renal-artery stenosis. N Engl J Med 2001;344:431–42.

[15] Sonpal GM, Sharma A, Miller A. Primary antiphospholipid antibody syndrome, renal infarction and hypertension. J Rheumatol 1993;20:1221–3.

[16] Peribasekar S, Chawla K, Rosner F, et al. Complete recovery from renal infarcts in a patient with mixed connective tissue disease. Am J Kidney Dis 1995;26:649–53.

[17] Godfrey T, Khamashta MA, Hughes GRV. Antiphospholipid syndrome and renal artery stenosis. Q J Med 2000;93:127–9.

[18] Aizawa K, Nakamura T, Sumino H, et al. Renovascular hypertension observed in a patient with antiphospholipid-antibodymsyndrome. Jpn Circ J 2000;64:541–3.

[19] Bhathena DB, Sobel BJ, Migdal SD. Non-inflammatory renal microangiopathy of systemic lupus erythematosus. ("lupus vaculitis"). Am J Nephrol 1981;1:144–59.

[20] Baldwin DS, Gluck MC, Lowenstein J, et al. Lupus nephritis: clinical course as related to morphological forms and their transitions. Am J Med 1977;62:12–30.

[21] Kleinknecht D, Bobrie G, Meyer O, et al. Recurrent thrombosis and renal vascular disease in patients with a lupus anticoagulant. Nephrol Dial Transplant 1989;4:854–8.

[22] Kincaid-Smith P, Fairley KF, Kloss M. Lupus anticoagulant associated with renal thrombotic microangiopathy and pregnancy-related renal failure. Q J Med 1988;69:795–815.

[23] Becquemont L, Thervet E, Rondeau E, et al. Systemic and renal fibrinolytic activity in a patient with anticardiolipin syndrome and renal thrombotic microangiopathy. Am J Nephrol 1990;10:254–8.

[24] D'Agati V, Kunis C, Williams G, et al. Anti-cardiolipin antibody and renal disease: a report of three cases. J Am Soc Nephrol 1990;1:777–84.

[25] Griffiths MH, Papadaki L, Neild GH. The renal pathology of primary antiphospholipid syndrome: a distinctive form of endothelial injury. Q J Med 2000;93:457–67.

[26] Ruggenenti P, Noria M, Remuzzi G. Thrombotic microangiopathy, haemolytic uremic syndrome, and thrombotic thrombocytopenic purpura. Kidney Int 2001;60:831–46.

[27] Erkan D, Cervera R, Asherson RA. Catastrophic antiphospholipid syndrome. Where do we stand? Arthritis Rheum 2003;48:3320–7.

[28] Wilkowski M, Arroyo R, McCabe K. Glomerulonephritis in a patient with anticardiolipin antibody. Am J Kidney Dis 1990;15:184–6.

[29] Almeshari K, Alfurayh O, Akhtar M. Primary antiphospholipid syndrome and self-limited renal vasculitis during pregnancy: case report and review of the literature. Am J Kidney Dis 1994;24:505–8.

[30] Fakhouri F, Noel LH, Zuber J, et al. The expanding spectrum of renal diseases associated with antiphospholipid syndrome. Am J Kidney Dis 2003;41:1205–11.

[31] Saracino A, Ramunni A, Pannarale G, et al. Kidney disease associated with primary antiphospholipid syndrome: clinical signs and histopathological features in an experience of five cases. Clin Nephrol 2005;63:471–6.

[32] Branch DW, Rodgers GM. Induction of endothelial cell tissue factor activity by sera from patients with antiphospholipid syndrome: a possible mechanism for thrombosis. Am J Obstet Gynecol 1993;168:206–10.

[33] Hamidou MA, Moreau A, Jego P, et al. Captopril and aspirin in the treatment of renal microangiopathy in primary antiphospholipid syndrome. Am J Kidney Dis 1995;25:486–8.

[34] Olguín L, Calleja C, Hernández C, et al. Primary antiphospholipid síndrome nephropathy despite anticoagulant therapy. Artritis Rheum 2003;48(Suppl):S359.

[35] Korkmaz C, Kabukcuoglu S, Isiksoy S, et al. Renal involvement in primary antiphospholipid syndrome and its response to immunosuppressive therapy. Lupus 2003;12:760–5.

[36] Bhowmik D, Dadhwal V, Dinda AK, et al. Steroid-responsive focal segmental glomerulosclerosis in primary antiphospholipid syndrome with successful pregnancy outcome. Nephrol Dial Transplant 2005;20:1726–8.

[37] Glueck HI, Kant KS, Weiss MA, et al. Thrombosis in systemic lupus erythematosus. Relation to the presence of circulating anticoagulants. Arch Intern Med 1985;145:1389–95.

[38] Liano F, Mampaso F, García Martín F. Allograft membranous glomerulonephritis and renal vein thrombosis in a patient with a lupus anticoagulant factor. Nephrol Dial Transplant 1988;3:684–9.

[39] Morgan RJ, Feneley CL. Renal vein thrombosis caused by primary antiphospholipid syndrome. Br J Urol 1994;74:807–8.

[40] Asherson RA, Buchanan N, Baguley E, et al. Postpartum bilateral renal vein thrombosis in the primary antiphospholipid syndrome. J Rheumatol 1993;20:874–6.

[41] Asherson RA, Lanham JG, Hull RG, et al. Renal vein thrombosis in systemic lupus associated with the lupus anticoagulant. Clin Exp Rheumatol 1984;2:47–51.

[42] Kant KS, PollaK VE, Weiss MA, et al. Glomerular thrombosis in systemic lupus erythematosus: Prevalence and significance. Medicine 1981;60:71–86.

[43] Moroni G, Ventura D, Riva P, et al. Antiphospholipid antibodies are associated with an increased risk for chronic renal insufficiency in patients with lupus nephritis. Am J Kidney Dis 2004;43:28–36.

[44] Miranda JM, García-Torres R, Jara LJ, et al. Renal biopsy in systemic lupus erythematosus: significance of glomerular trombosis. Analysis of 108 cases. Lupus 1994;3:25–9.

[45] Tektonidou MG, Sotsiou F, Nakopoulou L, et al. Antiphospholipid syndrome nephropathy in patients with systemic lupus erythematosus and antiphospholipid antibodies. Prevalence, clinical associations, and long-term outcome. Arthritis Rheum 2004;50:2569–79.

[46] Quereda C, Pardo A, Lamas S, et al. Lupus-like in vitro anticoagulant activity in end-stage renal disease. Nephron 1988;49:39–44.

[47] Gronhagen-Riska C, Teppo AM, Helantera A, et al. Raised concentrations of antibodies to cardiolipin in patients receiving dialysis. BMJ 1990;300:1696–7.

[48] Sitter T, Spannal M, Schiffl H. Anticardiolipin antibodies and lupus anticoagulant in patients treated with different methods of renal replacement therapy compared to patients with systemic lupus erythematosus. An epiphenomenon? Nephron 1993;64:655–6.

[49] García Martin F, De Arriba G, Carrascosa T, et al. Anticardiolipin antibodies and lupus anticoagulant in end-stage renal disease. Nephrol Dial Transpl 1991;6:543–7.

[50] Quereda C, Otero GG, Pordo A, et al. Prevalence of antiphospholipid antibodies in nephropaties not due to systemic lupus arythematosus. Am J Kidney Dis 1994;23:555–61.

[51] Brunet P, Aillaud M, San Marco M, et al. Antiphospholipids in hemodialysis patients. Relationship between lupus anticoagulant and thrombosis. Kid Int 1995;48:794–800.

[52] Fastenau DR, Wagenknecht DR, McIntyre JA. Increased incidence of antiphospholipid antibodies in left ventricular assist system recipients. Ann Thorac Surg 1999;68:137–42.

[53] Gharavi AE, Pierangeli S. Origin of antiphospholipid antibodies: induction by viral peptides. Lupus 1998;7(Suppl 2):S52–4.

[54] Matsuda J, Saitoh N, Gohchi K, et al. Beta 2-Glycoprotein-1-dependent and independent anticardiolipin antibody in patients with end-stage renal disease. Thromb Res 1993;72:109–17.

[55] Sitter T, Spannagl M, Schiffl H. Anticardiolipin antibodies and lupus anticoagulant in patients treated with different methods of renal replacement therapy in comparison to patients with systemic lupus erythematosus. Ann Hematol 1992;65:79–82.

[56] Phillips AO, Jones HW, Hambley H, et al. Prevalence of lupus anticoagulant and anticardiolipin antibodies in dialysis patients. Nephron 1993;65:350–3.

[57] Chew SL, Lins RL, Daelemans R, et al. Are antiphospholipid antibodies clinically relevant in dialysis patients? Nephrol Dial Transp 1992;14:1194–8.

[58] Fabrizi F, Sangiorgio R, Pontoriero G, et al. Antiphospholipid (APL) antibodies in end-stage renal disease. J Nephrol 1999;12:89–94.

[59] Prieto LN, Suki WN. Frequent hemodialysis graft thrombosis: association with antiphospholipid antibodies. Am J Kidney Dis 1994;23:587–90.

[60] Prakash R, Miller CC, Suki W. Anticardiolipin antibody in patients on maintenance hemodialysis and its association with recurrent arteriovenous graft thrombosis. Am J Kidney Dis 1995;26:347–52.

[61] Haviv YS. Association of anticardiolipin antibodies with vascular access occlusion in hemodialysis patients: cause or effect? Nephron 2000;86:447–54.

[62] Lesar CJ, Merrick HW, Smith MR. Thrombotic complications resulting from hypercoagulable states in chronic hemodialysis vascular access. J Am Coll Sur 1999;189:73–9.

[63] Yotsueda H, Tsuruya K, Tokumoto M, et al. Catastrophic antiphospholipid antibody syndrome following initiation of hemodialysis. Clin Exp Nephrol 2005;9:335–9.

[64] Stone JH, Amend WJC, Criswell LA. Outcome of renal transplantation in ninety-seven cyclosporine-era patients with systemic lupus erythematosus and matched controls. Arthritis Rheum 1998;41:1438–45.

[65] Radhakrishnan J, Williams GS, Appel GB, et al. Renal transplantation in anticardiolipin antibody-positive lupus erythematosus patients. Am J Kidney Dis 1994;23:286–9.

[66] Stone JH, Amend WJC, Criswell LA. Antiphospholipid antibody syndrome in renal transplantation: occurrence of clinical events in 96 consecutive patients with systemic lupus erythematosus. Am J Kidney Dis 1999;34:1040–7.

[67] Mondragón-Ramírez G, Bochicchio T, García-Torres R, et al. Recurrent renal thrombotic angiopathy after kidney transplantation in two patients with primary antiphospholipid syndrome (PAPS). Clin Transplant 1994;8:93–6.

[68] Vaidya S, Wang CC, Gugliuzza C, et al. Relative risk of post-transplant renal thrombosis in patients with antiphospholipid antibodies. Clin Transplant 1998;12:439–44.

[69] Vaidya S, Sellers R, Kimball P. Frequency, potential risk and therapeutic intervention in end-stage renal disease patients with antiphospholipid antibody syndrome: a multicenter study. Transplantation 2000;69:1348–52.

[70] Vaidya S, Gugliuzza K, Daller J. Efficacy of anticoagulation therapy in end-stage renal disease patients with antiphospholipid antibody syndrome. Transplantation 2004;77:1046–9.

[71] Baid Seema, Pascual M, Williams WW Jr, et al. Renal thrombotic micorangiopathy associated with anticardiolipin antibodies in hepatitis C-positive renal allograft recipients. J Am Soc Nephrol 1999;10:146–53.

ELSEVIER
SAUNDERS

Rheum Dis Clin N Am
32 (2006) 523–535

RHEUMATIC
DISEASE CLINICS
OF NORTH AMERICA

Osteoarticular Manifestations
of Antiphospholipid Syndrome

Maria G. Tektonidou, MD, PhD*,
Haralampos M. Moutsopoulos, MD, FACP, FRCP

*Department of Pathophysiology, Medical School, National University of Athens,
75 Mikras Asias str, Athens 11527, Greece*

Antiphospholipid syndrome (APS) is characterized by recurrent thromboses, pregnancy morbidity, and the presence of antiphospholipid antibodies (aPL), namely anticardiolipin antibodies (aCL) or lupus anticoagulant (LA) [1,2]. The sundrome is recognized as primary, or it can be associated with other underlying disorders, especially systemic lupus erythematosus (SLE). Thrombosis in APS may occur at any vascular site, and almost every organ system can be affected. However, osteoarticular manifestations in APS have been poorly recognized. Arthralgias represent the most commonly described musculoskeletal manifestations of primary and secondary APS, while arthritis has been primarily reported in SLE-related APS. Osteonecrosis has been described in association with aPL in patients with SLE or APS, as well as in several patients with nonautoimmune disorders.

Arthralgias and arthritis

Arthralgias are frequently reported in primary APS as well as in secondary APS; however, arthritis is mainly described in SLE-related APS patients. In the largest cohort of 1000 APS patients, 38.7% of patients had arthralgias, with a similar distribution among primary and secondary APS [2]. Weber and colleagues [3] reported that arthralgias or arthritis was documented in 83% of SLE-related APS versus 41% of primary APS patients, and emphasized the difficulty to distinguish frank and sustained arthritis from arthralgias on the basis of patient's history. Asherson and

---

* Corresponding author.
E-mail address: balts@otenet.gr (M.G. Tektonidou).

colleagues [4] noted that patients with primary APS do not have any of features closely related with SLE such as frank arthritis, serositis, vasculitic rash, or immune complex nephritis. Frank arthritis has also been included in the set of empirical exclusion criteria to distinguish primary APS from SLE-related APS, suggested by Piette and colleagues [5]. Queyrel and colleagues [6] described eight primary APS patients with nonerosive arthritis; nevertheless, they noted that three of them had lupus-like disease. In the multicentre study of 1000 APS individuals the prevalence of arthritis in SLE-related APS was 56% compared with only 3% in patients with primary APS [2]. Hence, it seems that arthritis is primarily observed in SLE or lupus-like patients with APS [4,7].

In primary APS, the treatment of arthralgias or arthritis includes the use of analgesics or nonsteroidal antinflammatory agents. These drugs should be used with caution in APS patients receiving chronic anticoagulant treatment because their combination has been associated with increased risk for bleeding complications. Corticosteroids, hydroxychloroquine, or other immunosuppressive drugs can also be used in patients with SLE-related APS, depending on the severity of articular symptoms or lupus activity.

Osteonecrosis

Osteonecrosis, or avascular necrosis, is a disease in which cell death in components of bone occurs as a result of blood supply interruption. Osteonecrosis has been associated with traumatic or other etiologic factors such as corticosteroids, alcoholism, sickle cell disease, pregnancy, or pancreatitis. If the etiology of osteonecrosis cannot be identified, the disease is classified as idiopathic. Multiple theories have been proposed regarding osteonecrosis pathogenesis such as mechanical vascular interruption (trauma, fractures), injury to or pressure on a vessel wall (vasculitis, Gaucher disease), embolism (by fat, nitrogen bubbles, sickle cells), and thrombosis or venous occlusion [8]. Thrombosis and ischemia has been first recognized as the predominant mechanism resulting to aseptic necrosis by Phemister in 1934 [9]. In 1974, Jones and colleagues [10] suggested that intravascular coagulation with fibrin thrombi represents the final pathway for osteonecrosis of various etiologies. Since then, the possible role of coagulation abnormalities in the pathogenesis of avascular necrosis has been widely examined in patients with or without autoimmune disorders. Idiopathic osteonecrosis of jaw in adults and Legg-Calve-Perthes disease in children has been associated with several acquired or inherited thrombophilic factors including protein C, S, or antithrombin III deficiency, activated protein C resistance, factor V Leiden, homocysteinemia and aPL, as well as with abnormal fibrinolysis [11–19]. In addition, histologic examinations in cases with nontraumatic osteonecrosis revealed thrombosis of terminal arteries in the subchondral bone [20]. Systematic evaluation of coagulation and fibrinolysis abnormalities for all patients diagnosed with osteonecrosis was proposed by several authors. aPL are associated with thromboses at vessels of all sizes, and they may play an important role in osteonecrosis development promoting thrombotic vasculopathy in the intraosseous microcirculation.

Osteonecrosis and antiphospholipid antibodies

Idiopathic osteonecrosis and antiphospholipid antibodies

An association between osteonecrosis and the presence of aPL has been documented in several cases with idiopathic osteonecrosis of the jaw and femoral head. Alijotas and colleagues [21] reported a series of 16 patients with Kienbock's disease (lunate osteonecrosis), and found that three patients had positive aCL; two of them had both aCL and LA. In a study by Glueck and colleagues [22], 43 of 55 patients with idiopathic osteonecrosis had one or more positive tests for thrombophilia or hypofibrinolysis; eight (33%) of 55 patients were aCL positive. Gruppo and colleagues [23] documented the presence of aCL in 18 (33%) of 55 patients with idiopathic avascular necrosis of the jaw. Korompilias and colleagues [24] examined 40 patients with nontraumatic osteonecrosis of the femoral head and found positive tests for IgG, IgM, or IgA aCL in 37.5% of patients. In a recent study [25], 37 (82%) of 45 patients with osteonecrosis (five with idiopathic) were found to have at least one coagulopathy versus 30% of controls ($P < 0.0001$). All five idiopathic patients had at least one coagulation factor abnormality; elevated aCL IgG were detected in four patients.

Human immunodeficiency virus infection and antiphospholipid antibodies

Avascular necrosis has been reported in several studies with human immunodeficiency virus (HIV) patients, occurring frequently in multiple sites and early in the course of disease. Rademaker and colleagues [26] reported six patients with HIV infection and avascular necrosis of multiple sites in the absence of known risk factors for osteonecrosis. Gerster and colleagues [27] suggested that the presence of unexplained multiple-site osteonecrosis should prompt consideration of HIV testing. During the last decade, a strong association has been documented between osteonecrosis and aPL in HIV-infected patients [28–35]. Olive and colleagues [33] reported four cases with hip osteonecrosis in a cohort of 1920 patients with HIV syndrome; three of them (75%) had positive aCL. Recently, Calza and colleagues [34] described seven HIV-infected persons with femoral head involvement. Among them, four patients were on antiretroviral therapy, one had moderate hypertriglyceridemia, and three were aCL positive. In another recent study [35], 339 asymptomatic HIV-infected adults were examined prospectively by magnetic resonance imaging (MRI) for osteonecrosis of the hip. Fifteen (4.4%) of 339 participants had osteonecrosis, and of these 14 (93%) had detectable levels of aCL.

Nevertheless, the association between osteonecrosis and aCL in patients with HIV infection should be interpreted with caution because these antibodies can be found in 80% to 90% of HIV-infected patients [36,37], and additionally, osteonecrosis has also been described in aCL-negative patients [27,38,39]. HIV itself and hypertriglyceridemia secondary to protease inhibitor treatment have also been implicated in the pathogenesis of osteonecrosis [40]; however, the first cases of osteonecrosis in HIV patients were reported before protease inhibitors became available [27,29]. Hence, the presence of aPL could be an additional risk factor for the development of osteonecrosis in HIV-infected patients, but further prospective studies with larger numbers of patients are needed to confirm this hypothesis.

Systemic lupus erythematosus and antiphospholipid antibodies

Osteonecrosis, in association with aCL, was first reported by Asherson and colleagues in 1985, in five patients with SLE [41]. One year later, Lavilla and colleagues [42] reported two other SLE patients with osteonecrosis and positive aCL. Nagasawa and colleagues [43], and later Mok and colleagues [44], showed an increased risk for osteonecrosis in SLE patients who were positive for LA. Abeles and colleagues [45] described a higher prevalence of aCL in SLE patients with osteonecrosis in comparison with those without osteonecrosis (35% versus 4%, $P = 0.008$). In 1993, Asherson and coolleagues [46] found that 27 (73%) of 37 SLE patients with symptomatic osteonecrosis had positive aPL. Mont and colleagues [47] found an association between osteonecrosis and IgM aCL, thrombophlebitis, mean corticosteroid dose, and vasculitis in lupus patients.

However, the correlation between avascular necrosis and aPL in SLE patients was not confirmed by other studies, suggesting different risk factors for osteonecrosis. Alarcon-Segovia and colleagues [48] failed to detect any association between osteonecrosis and aCL in a cohort of 500 consecutive SLE patients. Pistiner and colleagues [49] reported the presence of osteonecrosis in 26 (5.3%) of 488 SLE patients, and they noticed no correlation between bone necrosis and aCL. Migliaresi and colleagues [50] noted an association between osteonecrosis and continuous high-dose steroid treatment but not with serum levels of aCL. Petri and colleagues [51] described a significant association between osteonecrosis and Raynaud's phenomenon, vasculitis, and daily corticosteroid dosage, but not with aCL or LA. No correlation between avascular necrosis of the femoral head and aPL was detected in the studies by Dromer and colleagues [52] and Cozen and colleagues [53]. In another study [54] of 280 SLE patients no increased frequency of aPL, Raynaud's phenomenon, leukopenia, or SLE activity was found in patients with osteonecrosis compared with those without. Houssiau and colleagues [55] examined prospectively by MRI the presence of avascular necrosis in 40 SLE patients, and found that osteonecrosis was correlated only with corticosteroid use. Recently, Mok and colleagues [56] found no relationship between aCL or LA and the development of osteonecrosis in a cohort of 265 SLE patients followed for 20 years.

The controversy regarding the association between osteonecrosis and aPL is probably due to several methodologic characteristics of the above studies. Most of these series were retrospective, and they examined mainly symptomatic patients. However, it is well known that osteonecrosis can be entirely asymptomatic, and several subclinical cases may remain undiagnosed. The diagnosis of osteonecrosis in the majority of series was based on plain radiography, a method with limited sensitivity, especially in early stages. Moreover, almost all of the examined SLE patients were on corticosteroid treatment, which represents a significant predisposing factor for avascular necrosis. In addition, the laboratory methods for aPL measurement (commercial or home-made ELISA), the cutoff points, and the frequency of aPL positivity (once or on repeated measurements) varied among the studies.

Osteonecrosis and antiphospholipid syndrome

In most of the above studies examining the presence of osteonecrosis in SLE, the patients were divided to those with or without aPL without specifying if they fulfilled criteria for APS. In a retrospective study, Weber and colleagues [3] analyzed the data from 108 APS patients followed from 1987 to 1996. They reported that symptomatic osteonecrosis was found in 7 (10%) of 69 patients with secondary APS but in none of 22 patients with primary APS. In a European multicenter study [2] including 1000 patients with primary and secondary APS, the prevalence of symptomatic osteonecrosis was 2.4%.

In the above studies, the majority of SLE-related APS patients were on corticosteroid treatment. Corticosteroid therapy is widely used in SLE-related APS patients, but rather rarely in patients with primary APS. The presence of osteonecrosis in primary APS in the absence of steroid use suggests an association between APS and osteonecrosis (Table 1). The existence of osteonecrosis in primary APS patients not receiving corticosteroids was first documented by Asherson and colleagues [4]. The authors found that 2 out of 70 studied patients had symptomatic osteonecrosis, which was the initial manifestation of the syndrome in one of them. Alijotas and colleagues [21] reported the presence of aPL in 3 of 16 patients with Kienbocks disease; one of them had a history of deep vein thrombosis and recurrent abortions in association with positive aCL and LA. Vela and colleagues [57] described a patient with primary APS who suffered a previous deep vein thrombosis and subsequently developed osteonecrosis of the hip. Similarly, a patient with a history of hemiplegic migraine and cerebrovascular infarcts who developed osteonecrosis of the left hip and the right knee has been also reported [58]. Dubost [59] documented a case with fatal primary APS and multiple bone necrotic areas. Regarding catastrophic APS, Egan and

Table 1
Patients with primary APS and osteonecrosis in the absence of corticosteroid use

Authors	Study design	Number of patients with osteonecrosis	Osteonecrosis site	LA	aCL
Asherson et al (1989) [53]	Cross-sectional	2/70	NR	NR	NR
Alijotas et al (1990) [4]	Case series	1/16	Lunate	+	+
Vela et al (1991) [57]	Case report	1	Femoral head	+	−
Seleznick et al (1991) [58]	Case report	1	Femoral head, knee	−	+
Egan et al (1991) [60]	Case report	1	Multifocal	+	+
Dubost et al (1994) [59]	Case report	1	Femoral head, knee, humerus	+	+
Tektonidou et al (2003) [62]	Prospective	6/30	Femoral head	3+/3−	+

Abbreviations: aCL, anticardiolipin antibodies; LA, lupus anticoagulant; NR, not reported.

colleagues [60] described a 25-year-old woman who presented with hemo-lytic anemia, thrombocytopenia, renal insufficiency, and multiple sites of thrombosis and osteonecrosis. In a series of 80 patients with catastrophic APS, symptomatic osteonecrosis was found in 7% of cases [61].

Recently, we examined prospectively by MRI 30 asymptomatic patients with primary APS, 19 SLE patients (9 with positive aPL, 10 with negative aPL), and 30 healthy individuals for hip osteonecrosis. All the patients had never received steroid treatment [62]. Osteonecrosis was diagnosed in 6 (20%) of 30 APS patients but in none of SLE patients or healthy controls. Three patients had early osteonecrosis (bilateral in one patient), and three had established bilateral osteonecrosis. Early osteonecrosis was indicated by a band or rim in the subchondral zone with decreased intensity signal on both T1- and T2-weighted images (band sign), while established osteo-necrosis by the characteristic double-line sign (Figs. 1 and 2). Osteonecrosis in our study occurred significantly more frequently in younger patients and in those with livedo reticularis (Fig. 3).

Livedo reticularis represents the most common skin manifestation of APS, characterized by diminished blood flow in arterioles and dilatation of venules and capillaries. In a recent study by Francès and colleagues [63], livedo reticularis was found to be strongly associated with arterial events in APS, and it was suggested as a strong marker of arterial/arteriolar APS subset. The association between osteonecrosis and livedo reticularis in APS patients suggests that microvasculopathy may be the underlying mech-anism for osteonecrosis development. In addition, Hatzigeorgiou and col-leagues [64] found a high frequency (57%) of cerebral white matter lesions (WML) in patients with nontraumatic osteonecrosis of the femoral head. The pathogenesis of WML remains largely unknown, but it is generally thought that WML are related to cerebral microvascular disease. WML have been associated with age and the presence of vascular risk factors such as hypertension, stroke, diabetes, hyperlipidemia, and smoking. No

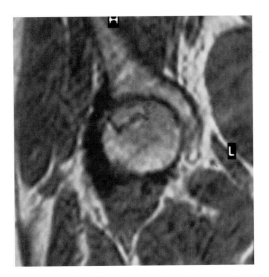

Fig. 1. Early osteonecrosis on this T1-weighted spin echo magnetic resonance is indicated by the low-intensity band in the subchondral zone of the femoral head (band sign). This image displays an osteonecrosis area with fat like signal, involving no more than 25% of the weight-bearing surface of the femoral head.

relationship between WML and steroid use, hyperlipidemia, or other risk factors was described in the above study. The association between osteonecrosis and WML gives further support to the role of microangiopathy in avascular necrosis pathogenesis.

Clinical manifestations of osteonecrosis

The blood supply to the humeral and femoral head, talus, and carpal bones are critical to the development of osteonecrosis at these sites. The femoral head represents the most vulnerable site for the development of osteonecrosis. The clinical manifestations of osteonecrosis depend on the stage of the disease and the site of involvement. Osteonecrosis is usually asymptomatic, especially in early stages. If present, localized pain and movement limitation is the most common presentation of bone infarcts. In some cases, atypical sites of osteonecrosis have been described affecting a single vertebral body, lunate bone, or ribs [21,65,66]. Multiple sites of bones can also be involved, especially in SLE patients [67,68].

Diagnosis and treatment of osteonecrosis

Plain radiography has limited sensitivity in the diagnosis of early osteonecrosis. However, the pathognomonic subchondral radiolucent line (crescent sign), bone collapse or fractures, sclerosis, and periostitis can be detected in established osteonecrosis [69]. CT scans is not as sensitive as

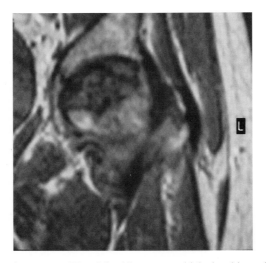

Fig. 2. Double-line sign seen on T1-weighted images as a high-signal intensity line in an inner zone combined with low-signal intensity in an outer zone involving more than 50% of the weight-bearing surface of the femoral head. Irregularity of the articular surface is also detected.

radionuclide imaging or MRI. MRI represents the most sensitive method for the diagnosis of osteonecrosis with an overall sensitivity of more than 95% [70,71]. The earliest finding on MRI is a density line (low intensity signal) that represents the separation of normal and ischemic bone. The most characteristic finding is the double-line sign seen as a high signal intensity line in an inner zone combined with low-signal intensity in an outer zone on T2-weighted images and less frequently on T1-images.

The treatment of osteonecrosis depends on the location, site, and stage of the lesion. Early diagnosis is crucial in preventing or arresting the disease process. Other associated conditions such as infections (osteomyelitis) or

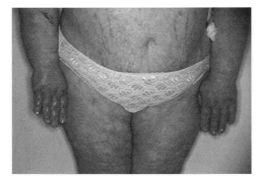

Fig. 3. Livedo reticularis in a woman with primary APS and osteonecrosis of the femoral head.

tumors in the affected site should be ruled out. In early stages, a conservative treatment is recommended, including steroid tapering, use of analgesics, bed rest, and weight-bearing avoidance. Several surgical approaches have been tried with variable success. Core decompression with or without bone grafting or osteotomies are indicated in early stages [72,73]. In late stages, total joint arthroplasty is the surgical treatment of choice [74].

Orthopedic surgery and particularly hip replacement has a high risk of postoperative thrombosis. Patients with APS are at significantly increased risk of postoperative thrombotic complications due to increased hypercoaguability, warfarin withdrawal, or development of catastrophic APS triggered by the surgical procedure. Thus, a proper perioperative medical management of these patients during orthropedic procedures is mandatory. The main goal of the treatment protocols is the minimization of periods without anticoagulation and the use of the appropriate anticoagulant doses to avoid both thrombotic and life-threatening bleeding complications [75,76]. Warfarin treatment is usually discontinued 3 to 4 days before surgery, and low molecular weight heparin or intravenous heparin is administered during perioperative period. Warfarin can be reinstituted some days or 2 to 4 weeks after surgical procedure, depending on the risk of bleeding [75,76].

Besides the above surgical procedures, the use of anticoagulant treatment in aPL-positive patients with early osteonecrosis should also be examined in large, prospective studies.

Nontraumatic fractures

Sangle and colleagues [77] described 19 aPL-positive patients with SLE who presented with foot pain. All of them had metatarsal fractures (six bilaterally) without any obvious history of trauma. Seventeen of 19 patients had APS, most of them in the context of SLE. Five patients had osteoporosis and one had osteopenia. The authors suggested that bone microinfarcts may lead to bone damage and fractures in patients with positive aPL.

Bone marrow necrosis

Bone marrow necrosis is defined morphologically by destruction of hematopoietic tissue, including the stroma, with preservation of the bone. It has been associated with several conditions including sickle cell disease, acute leukemia, metastatic neoplasia, and bacterial infection, as well as disseminated intravascular coagulation following irradiation and antineoplastic therapy. The association between bone marrow necrosis and APS has been first reported by Bulvik and colleagues [78]. Since then, several other cases have been published, some of them with fatal outcome in the context of catastrophic APS [79–84]. Asherson and colleagues [61] described a 7%

prevalence of bone marrow necrosis among 80 patients with catastrophic APS.

Summary

In conclusion, arthralgias represent a rather common osteoarticular manifestation of primary and secondary APS, while arthritis is mainly described in SLE-related APS. Osteonecrosis is frequently described in association with aPL in patients with and without autoimmune disorders. The presence of osteonecrosis in primary APS patients in the absence of corticosteroid use suggests an association between osteonecrosis and APS. Clinicians should be aware of this possible clinical manifestation of APS, because early diagnosis may lead to early management. A systematic screening for aPL in all cases with diagnosed osteonecrosis in the absence of precipitating factors should be considered.

References

[1] Hughes GR. The antiphospholipid syndrome: ten years on. Lancet 1993;342(8867):341–4.

[2] Cervera R, Piette JC, Font J, et al. Antiphospholipid syndrome: clinical and immunological manifestations and patterns of disease expression in a cohort of 1000 patients. Arthritis Rheum 2002;46(4):1019–27.

[3] Weber M, Hayem G, de Bandt M, et al. Classification of an intermediate group of patients with antiphospholipid syndrome and lupus-like disease: primary or secondary antiphospholipid syndrome? J Rheumatol 1999;26:2131–6.

[4] Asherson RA, Khamashta MA, Ordi-Ros J, et al. "Primary" antiphospholipid syndrome: major clinical and serological features. Medicine (Baltimore) 1989;68(6):366–74.

[5] Piette JC, Whechsler B, Francès C, et al. Exclusion criteria for primary antiphospholipid syndrome. J Rheumatol 1993;20(10):1802–3.

[6] Queyrel V, Hachula E, Cardon T. Arthritis in primary antiphospholipid syndrome? J Rheumatol 1996;23(7):1305.

[7] Piette JC, Asherson RA. Arthritis in primary antiphospholipid syndrome? Reply. J Rheumatol 1996;23(7):1305–6.

[8] Mankin HJ. Nontraumatic necrosis of bone (osteonecrosis). N Engl J Med 1992;326(22): 1473–9.

[9] Phemister DB. Fractures of the neck of the femur, dislocation of hip, and obscure vascular disturbances producing aseptic necrosis of the head of the femur. Surg Gynec Obstet 1934; 59:415–40.

[10] Jones JP Jr, Sakovich L, Anderson CE. Experimentally produced osteonecrosis as a result of fat embolism. In: Beckman EL, Elliott DH, Smith EM, editors. Dysbarism-related osteonecrosis. HEW publ (NIOSH) 75-153. Washington (DC): U.S. Government Printing Office; 1974. p. 117–32.

[11] Boettcher WG, Bonfiglio M, Hamilton HH, et al. Nontraumatic necrosis of the femoral head. Relation of altered hemostasis to etiology. J Bone Joint Surg Am 1970;52(2):312–21.

[12] Glueck CJ, Glueck HI, Greenfield D, et al. Protein C and S deficiency, thrombophilia and hypofibrinolysis: pathophysiologic causes of Legg-Perthes disease. Pediatr Res 1994;35 (4 Pt1):383–8.

[13] Glueck CJ, Freiberg R, Tracy T, et al. Thrombophilia and hypofibrinolysis. Pathophysiologies of osteonecrosis. Clin Orthop 1997;334:43–56.

[14] Van Veldhuizen PJ, Neff J, Murphey M, et al. Decreased fibrinolytic potential in patients with idiopathic avascular necrosis and transient osteoporosis of the hip. Am J Hematol 1993;44(4):243–8.

[15] Arruda VR, Belangero WD, Ozelo MC, et al. Inherited risk factors for thrombophilia among children with Legg-Calve-Perthes disease. J Pediatr Orthop 1999;19(1):84–7.

[16] Glueck CJ, Crawford A, Roy D, et al. Association of antithrombotic factor deficiencies and hypofibrinolysis with Legg-Perthes disease. J Bone Joint Surg 1996;78(1):3–13.

[17] Balassa VV, Gruppo RA, Glueck CJ, et al. Legg-Calve-Perthes disease and thrombophilia. J Bone Joint Surg Am 2004;86-A(12):2642–7.

[18] Herndon WA. Association of antithrombotic factor deficiencies and hypofibrinolysis with Legg-Perthes disease. J Bone Joint Surg Am 1997;79(7):1114–5.

[19] Tektonidou MG, Moutsopoulos HM. Immunologic factors in the pathogenesis of osteonecrosis. Orthop Clin North Am 2004;35(3):259–63.

[20] Jones JP Jr. Intravascular coagulation and osteonecrosis. Clin Orthop 1992;277:41–53.

[21] Alijotas J, Argemi M, Barquinero J. Kienbock's disease and antiphospholipid antibodies. Clin Exp Rheumatol 1990;8(3):297–8.

[22] Glueck CJ, McMahon RE, Bouquot JE, et al. The pathophysiology of idiopathic osteonecrosis of the jaws: thrombophilia and hypofibrinolysis (abstract). J Invest Med 1995;43 (Suppl 2):234A.

[23] Gruppo R, Glueck CJ, McMahon RE. The pathophysiology of alveolar osteonecrosis of the jaw: anticardiolipin antibodies, thrombophilia and hypofibrinolysis. J Lab Clin Med 1996; 127(5):481–8.

[24] Korompilias AV, Gilkeson GS, Ortel TL, et al. Anticardiolipin antibodies and osteonecrosis of the femoral head. Clin Orthop 1997;345:174–80.

[25] Jones LC, Mont MA, Petri M, et al. Procoagulants and osteonecrosis. J Rheumatol 2003; 30(4):783–91.

[26] Rademaker J, Dobro JS, Solomon G. Osteonecrosis and human immunodeficiency virus infection. J Rheumatol 1997;24(3):601–4.

[27] Gerster JC, Camus JP, Chave JP, et al. Multiple site avascular necrosis in HIV infected patients. J Rheumatol 1991;18(2):300–2.

[28] Solomon G, Brancato L, Winchester R. An approach to the human immunodeficiency virus positive patient with a spondyloarthropathic disease. Rheum Dis Clin North Am 1991;17(1): 42–58.

[29] Chevalier X, Larget-Piet B, Hernigou P, et al. Avascular necrosis of te femoral head in HIV-infected patients. J Bone Joint Surg Br 1993;75(1):160.

[30] Belmonte MA, Garcia-Portales R, Domenech I, et al. Avascular necrosis of bone in human immunodeficiency virus infection and antiphospholipid antibodies. J Rheumatol 1993;20(8): 1425–8.

[31] Molina JF, Citera G, Rosler D. Coexistence of human immunodeficiency virus infection and systemic lupus erythematosus. J Rheumatol 1995;22(2):347–50.

[32] Koeger AC, Banneville B, Gerster JC, et al. Avascular osteonecrosis in HIV-infected patients: 10 cases (abstract 277). Arthritis Rheum 1995;38(Suppl):S119.

[33] Olive A, Queralt C, Sirera G, et al. Osteonecrosis and HIV-infection: 4 more cases. J Rheumatol 1998;25(6):1243–4.

[34] Calza L, Manfredi R, Chiodo F. Osteonecrosis in HIV-infected patients and its correlation with highly active antiretroviral therapy (HAART). Presse Med 2003;32(13 Pt 1):595–8.

[35] Miller KD, Masur H, Jones EC, et al. High prevalence of osteonecrosis of the femoral head in HIV-infected adults. Ann Intern Med 2002;137(1):17–25.

[36] Stimmler MM, Quismorio FP, McGehee WG, et al. Anticardiolipin antibodies in acquired immunodeficiency syndrome. Arch Intern Med 1989;149(8):1833–5.

[37] Coll Daroca J, Gutierrez-Cebollada J, Yazbeck H, et al. Anticardiolipin antibodies and acquired immunodeficiency syndrome. Prognostic marker or association with HIV infection. Infection 1992;20(3):140–2.

[38] Llauger J, Palmer J, Roson N, et al. Osteonecrosis of the knee in an HIV-infected patient. AJR Am J Roentgenol 1998;171(4):987–8.

[39] Johns DG, Gill MJ. Avascular necrosis in HIV infection. AIDS 1999;13(14):1997–8.

[40] Monier P, McKown K, Bronze MS. Osteonecrosis complicating highly active antiretroviral therapy in patients infected with human immunodeficiency virus. Clin Infect Dis 2000;31(6): 1488–92.

[41] Asherson RA, Jungers P, Liote F. Ischaemic necrosis of bone associated with the "lupus anticoagulant" and antibodies to cardiolipin [abstract]. In: Proceedings of the XVIth International Congress of Rheumatology, Sydney (Australia); 1985. p. 373.

[42] Lavilla P, Gil A, Khamashta MA, et al. Necrosis osea avasculary lupus eritematoso sistematico. Rev Clin Esp 1987;181(5):289–90.

[43] Nagasawa K, Ishii Y, Mayumi T, et al. Avascular necrosis of bone in systemic lupus erythematosus: possible role of haemostatic abnormalities. Ann Rheum Dis 1989;48(8): 672–6.

[44] Mok CC, Lau CS, Wong RW. Risk factors for avascular bone necrosis in systemic lupus erythematosus. Br J Rheumatol 1998;37(8):895–900.

[45] Abeles M, Urman JD, Rothfield NF. Aseptic necrosis of bone in systemic lupus erythematosus. Relation to corticosteroid therapy. Arch Intern Med 1978;138(5):750–75.

[46] Asherson RA, Liote F, Page B, et al. Avascular necrosis of bone and antiphospholipid antibodies in systemic lupus erythematosus. J Rheumatol 1993;20(2):284–8.

[47] Mont MA, Glueck CJ, Pacheco IH, et al. Risk factors for osteonecrosis in systemic lupus erythematosus. J Rheumatol 1997;24(4):654–62.

[48] Alarcon-Segovia D, Deleze M, Oria CV, et al. Antiphospholipid antibodies and the antiphospholipid syndrome in systemic lupus erythematosus. A prospective analysis of 500 consecutive patients. Medicine 1989;68(6):353–65.

[49] Pistiner M, Wallace DJ, Nessim S, et al. Lupus erythematosus in the 1980s: a survey of 570 patients. Sem Arthritis Rheum 1991;21(1):55–64.

[50] Migliaresi S, Picillo U, Ambrosone L, et al. Avascular osteonecrosis in patients with SLE: relation to corticosteroid therapy and anticardiolipin antibodies. Lupus 1994;3:37–41.

[51] Petri M. Muscosceletal complications of systemic lupus erythematosus in the Hopkins Lupus Cohort: an update. Arthritis Care Res 1995;8(3):137–45.

[52] Dromer C, Marc V, Laroche M, et al. No link between avascular necrosis of the femoral head and antiphospholipid antibodies. Rev Rhum Engl Ed 1997;64(6):382–5.

[53] Cozen L, Wallace DJ. Avascular necrosis in systemic lupus erythematosus: clinical associations and a 47-year perspective. Am J Orthop 1998;27(5):352–4.

[54] Rascu A, Manger K, Kraetsch HG, et al. Osteonecrosis in systemic lupus erythematosus, steroid induced or a lupus-dependent manifestation? Lupus 1996;5(4):323–7.

[55] Houssiau FA, N'Zeusseu Toukap A, Depresseux G, et al. Magnetic resonance imaging-detected avascular osteonecrosis in systemic lupus erythematosus: lack of correlation with antiphospholipid antibodies. Br J Rheumatol 1998;37(4):448–53.

[56] Mok MY, Farewell VT, Isenberg DA. Risk factors for avascular necrosis of bone in patients with systemic lupus erythematosus: is there a role for antiphospholipid antibodies? Ann Rheum Dis 2000;59(6):462–7.

[57] Vela P, Battle E, Salas E, et al. Primary antiphospholipid syndrome and osteonecrosis. Clin Exp Rheumatol 1991;9:545–6.

[58] Seleznick MJ, Silveira LH, Espinosa LR. Avascular necrosis associated with anticardiolipin antibodies. J Rheumatol 1991;18(9):1416–7.

[59] Dubost JJ, Kemeny JL, Soubrier M, et al. Primary antiphospholipid syndrome of fatal course and osteorticular cytosteatonecrosis. Rev Med Interne 1994;15(8):535–40.

[60] Egan RM, Munn RK. Catastrophic antiphospholipid antibody syndrome presenting with multiple thromboses and sites of avascular necrosis. J Rheumatol 1994;21(12):2376–9.

[61] Asherson RA, Cervera R, Piette JC, et al. Catastrophic antiphospholipid syndrome: clues to the pathogenesis from a series of 80 patients. Medicine 2001;80(6):355–77.

[62] Tektonidou MG, Malagari K, Vlachoyiannopoulos PG, et al. Asymptomatic avascular necrosis in patients with primary antiphospholipid syndrome in the absence of corticosteroid use: a prospective study by magnetic resonance imaging. Arthritis Rheum 2003;48(3):732–6.

[63] Frances C, Niang S, Laffite E, et al. Dermatologic manifestations of the antiphospholipid syndrome: two hundred consecutive cases. Arthritis Rheum 2005;52(6):1785–93.

[64] Hatjigeorgiou GM, Karantanas AH, Zibis A, et al. Increased frequency of white matter lesions in patients with osteonecrosis (WMLeOn) of the femoral head. Eur J Rad 2004;50(3): 278–84.

[65] Mok MY, Isenberg DA. Avascular necrosis of a single vertebral body, an atypical site of disease in a patient with SLE and secondary APLS. Ann Rheum Dis 2000;59(6):494.

[66] Yoo WH. Multiple rib infarcts: a rare form of osteonecrosis in antiphospholipid syndrome. Ann Rheum Dis 2004;63(4):457–8.

[67] Galindo M, Mateo I, Pablos JL. Multiple avascular necrosis of bone and polyarticular septic arthritis in patients with systemic lupus erythematosus. Rheumatol Int 2005;25(1):72–6.

[68] Fishel B, Caspi D, Eventov I, et al. Multiple osteonecrotic lesions in systemic lupus erythematosus. J Rheumatol 1987;14(3):601–4.

[69] Plakseychuk AY, Shah M, Varitimidis SE, et al. Classification of osteonecrosis of the femoral head. Reliability, reproducibility, and prognostic value. Clin Orthop Relat Res 2001; 386:34–41.

[70] Tervonen O, Mueller DM, Matteson EL, et al. Clinically occult avascular necrosis of the hip: prevalence in an asymptomatic population at risk. Radiology 1992;182(3):845–7.

[71] Coleman BG, Kressel HY, Dalinka MK, et al. Radiographically negative avascular necrosis: detection with MR imaging. Radiology 1988;168(2):525–8.

[72] Mont MA, Carbone JJ, Fairbank AC. Core decompression versus nonoperative management for osteonecrosis of the hip. Clin Orthop Rel Res 1996;324:169–78.

[73] D' Souza SR, Sadiq S, Northmore-Balle MD. Proximal femoral osteotomy as the primary operation for young adults who have osteoarthritis of the hip. J Bone Joint Surg 1998; 80A:1428–38.

[74] Cornell CN, Salvati EA, Pelicci PM. Long term follow-up of total hip replacement in patients with osteonecrosis. Orthop Clin North Am 1985;16(4):757–69.

[75] Vasoo S, Sangle S, Zain M, et al. Orthopaedic manifestations of the antiphospholipid (Hughes) syndrome. Lupus 2005;14(5):339–45.

[76] Erkan D, Leibowitz E, Berman J, et al. Perioperative medical management of antiphospholipid syndrome: hospital for special surgery experience, review of literature and recommendations. J Rheumatol 2002;29(4):843–9.

[77] Sangle S, D'Cruz D, Khamashta MA, et al. Antiphospholipid antibodies, systemic lupus erythematosus and non-traumatic metatarsal fractures. Ann Rheum Dis 2004;63(10):1241–3.

[78] Bulvik S, Aronson I, Ress S, et al. Extensive bone marrow necrosis associated with antiphospholipid antibodies. Am J Med 1995;98(6):572–4.

[79] Paydas S, Kocak R, Zorludemir S, et al. Bone marrow necrosis in antiphospholipid syndrome. J Clin Pathol 1997;50(3):261–2.

[80] Murphy PT, Sivakumaran M, Casey MC, et al. Lymphoma associated bone marrow necrosis with raised anticardiolipin antibody. J Clin Pathol 1998;51(5):407–9.

[81] Moore J, Ma DD, Concannon A. Non-malignant bone marrow necrosis: a report of two cases. Pathology 1998;30(3):318–20.

[82] Schaar CG, Ronday KH, Boets EP, et al. Catastrophic manifestation of the antiphospholipid syndrome. J Rheumatol 1999;26(10):2261–4.

[83] Thuerl C, Altehoefer C, Spyridonidis A, et al. Imaging findings in the rare catastrophic variant of the primary antiphospholipid syndrome. Eur Radiol 2002;12(3):545–8.

[84] Sinha J, Chowdhry I, Sedan S, et al. Bone marrow necrosis and refractory HELLP syndrome in a patient with catastrophic antiphospholipid antibody syndrome. J Rheumatol 2002; 29(1):195–7.

ELSEVIER
SAUNDERS

Rheum Dis Clin N Am
32 (2006) 537–551

RHEUMATIC
DISEASE CLINICS
OF NORTH AMERICA

Accelerated Atheroma in the Antiphospholipid Syndrome

Eiji Matsuura, PhD[a],*, Kazuko Kobayashi, PhD[a],
Masako Tabuchi, MD[a], Luis R. Lopez, MD[b]

[a]Department of Cell Chemistry, Okayama University, Graduate School of Medicine Dentistry
and Pharmaceutical Sciences, 2-5-1 Shikata-cho, Okayama 700-8558, Japan
[b]Corgenix, Inc., 12601 Tejon Street, Westminster, CO 80234, USA

Increased cardiovascular morbidity and mortality due to the premature or accelerated development of atherosclerosis has been reported in patients with systemic autoimmune diseases such as a systemic lupus erythematosus (SLE) [1–3]. These findings motivated a great deal of research into the role of autoimmunity in atherogenesis. The relationship of cholesterol metabolism to atherosclerosis has been well established. However, the participation of newer inflammatory and immunologic mechanisms are emerging as relevant factors for the initiation and progression of atherosclerotic lesions. The oxidative modification of low-density lipoprotein (oxLDL) with the development of autoantibodies to oxLDL have been identified as key pro-atherogenic events that accelerate the formation of macrophage-derived foam cells and atherosclerotic lesions [4–7]. Many of the life-threatening clinical complications presented by patients with antiphospholipid syndrome (APS) involve both the venous and arterial blood vessels. Since the original description of APS, much attention has been directed toward the basic and clinical mechanisms of vascular injury and thrombosis. The venous and arterial thromboembolic events of APS are associated with elevated serum levels of antiphospholipid antibodies, and frequently observed in the context of an autoimmune disorder [8,9]. The exact mechanism by which antiphospholipid antibodies promote thrombosis is not yet completely understood. However, it is widely accepted that these antibodies play a direct pathogenic role in the development of thrombosis. Venous thrombosis is the most common vascular event; however, one of three APS patients presents arterial thrombosis (myocardial infarction, cerobrovascular accident, angina, and

* Corresponding author.
E-mail address: eijimatu@md.okayama-u.ac.jp (E. Matsuura).

0889-857X/06/$ - see front matter © 2006 Elsevier Inc. All rights reserved.
doi:10.1016/j.rdc.2006.05.006

rheumatic.theclinics.com

so on) during the evolution of the disease [10–12]. Experimental evidence suggest that β_2-glycoprotein I (β_2GPI) is the major antigenic target for anti-phospholipid antibodies, and thought to play a central role in the development of the clinical complications of APS [13–16]. Further, anti-β_2GPI antibodies have been associated with the history of arterial thrombosis [17–19]. OxLDL is the principal lipoprotein found in atherosclerotic lesions by immunohistochemical analysis, and it colocalizes with β_2GPI, immunoreactive CD4 and CD8 lymphocytes and immunoglobulins [20,21]. These findings further suggested an active role of antiphospholipid antibodies in atherogenesis. OxLDL binds to β_2GPI in vitro, and circulating OxLDL/β_2GPI complexes were demonstrated in patients with various systemic autoimmune and chronic inflammatory diseases, such as SLE, APS, chronic renal disease, diabetes mellitus, and in some patients with acute myocardial infarction [22–25]. IgG antibodies to OxLDL/β_2GPI complexes were only detected in patients with SLE and APS, and were strongly associated with arterial thrombosis [26]. In vitro experiments have shown that OxLDL/β_2GPI complexes were more rapidly internalized by macrophages when anti-β_2GPI antibodies were present, suggesting the participation of Fcγ receptors [23–25]. Thus, circulating IgG immune complexes containing oxLDL and β_2GPI may be atherogenic.

Atherosclerosis and autoimmunity

Atherosclerosis is the most important underlying cause of cardiovascular morbidity and mortality in the general population. In the United States alone, over 61 million Americans have a form of cardiovascular disease; of these, 7.3 million had a myocardial infarction and 4.5 million a cerebrovascular accident. Complications from atherosclerotic disease are typically chronic, with high recurrence and mortality rates, claiming the lives of approximately half a million people each year [26]. The Framingham study identified the following risk factors for atherosclerosis: hypertension, hypercholesterolemia from either dietary or hereditary causes, diabetes mellitus, obesity, smoking, family history, and inactive lifestyles. These risk factors are thought to contribute to the initiation and progression of atherosclerosis by disrupting a number of lipid regulatory and inflammatory mechanisms within the arterial wall. The causal relationship between atherosclerosis and blood cholesterol has been well established. The cholesterol present in atherosclerotic lesions originates in the blood. Of the subclasses of cholesterol, low-density lipoprotein (LDL) is the main pro-atherogenic 4 subclass, but LDL has to be first modified to promote atherosclerosis [27,28]. oxLDL promotes inflammation attracting monocytes and T-lymphocytes to the lesion, is cytotoxic for endothelial cells causing a pro-thrombotic endothelial surface dysfunction, and stimulates the release of various soluble inflammatory and adhesion molecules. In addition to proinflammatory properties, oxLDL is also highly immunogenic [29,30]. Anti-oxLDL antibodies have been detected in individuals with atherosclerotic cardiovascular diseases [31,32]. Although most of the atherosclerotic changes occur inside the arterial wall, there is also an endothelial and platelet pro-thrombotic dysfunction that leads to increased arterial thrombois when plaques become unstable and rupture. The term atherothrombosis more appropriately describes the late occurrence of arterial thrombosis in complicated atherosclerosis. All these findings suggested a complex interrelationship between dyslipoproteinemia, inflammation, and immunologic mechanisms, sharply contrasting with the purely metabolic or passive origin of atherosclerosis initially proposed. The premature development of atherosclerosis has been recently reported in patients with systemic autoimmune diseases [1,2]. The traditional Framingham risk factors as well as anti-inflammatory or immunosuppressive therapeutic programs (ie, steroids) failed to fully account for the accelerated development of atherosclerosis in patients with SLE [33]. With today's 10-year survival rate of over 80%, new causes of SLE morbidity and mortality have emerged. Mortality rates due to cardiovascular disease have surpassed that from the SLE disease itself or from complications such as infections [3]. The prevalence of symptomatic coronary heart disease in SLE ranges from 6% to 15%, with an overall incidence of myocardial infarction five times higher than the general population. When adjusted to age, the incidence of myocardial infarction can be as high as 50 times. In addition, 43% of asymptomatic SLE patients had abnormal myocardial perfusion results by Tc99m emission tomography, and over 33% had increased carotid intima-media thickness with atherosclerotic plaques demonstrated by B-mode ultrasound.

Atherosclerosis and antiphospholipid syndrome

APS is the most common cause of acquired hypercoagulability in the general population [34,35]. Elevated serum levels of antiphospholipid antibodies along with thromboembolic complications involving both the venous and arterial blood vessels, or with pregnancy morbidity (miscarriages and fetal loss) represent the major features of APS. If APS is present in patients with an underlying systemic autoimmune disorder, that is SLE, is referred to as secondary APS, but if present in the absence of an obvious underlying disease is referred to as primary APS [8]. Antiphospholipid antibodies increase the risk of thrombosis by at least twofold when present in the context of an autoimmune disease [36]. In both primary and secondary APS, recurrence rates of up to 30% for thrombosis with a mortality of up to 10% over a 10-year follow-up period have been reported [37,38]. Venous thromboembolic events represent the most common clinical finding in patients with APS [10]. However, about 25% of APS patients enrolled into a European cohort of 1000 patients presented an arterial thrombotic event (myocardial infarction, cerebrovascular accident, angina, and so on) as the initial clinical manifestation. If all the initial and late arterial thrombotic events were considered, up to

31% of the patients developed these complications [39]. These observations not only support the hypothesis of autoimmune mechanism(s), but suggest a role of antiphospholipid antibodies in atherosclerosis.

Vascular inflammation in autoimmune diseases may cause oxidation of LDL and the interaction of oxLDL with various plasma proteins including β_2GPI. These events may favor the production of autoantibodies which in turn, would accelerate the development of venous and arterial thrombosis. Antiphospholipid antibodies (anticardiolipin antibodies [aCL] or lupus anticoagulants) are a heterogeneous group of autoantibodies characterized by their reactivity to negatively charged phospholipids, phospholipid/protein complexes, and certain proteins presented on appropriate surfaces (ie, activated cell membranes, oxygenated polystyrene) [11]. Plasma proteins that participate in blood coagulation and interact with phospholipids have been described as antiphospholipid cofactors, that is, β_2GPI, prothrombin, annexin V. β_2GPI has been shown to be a relevant antigenic target for antiphospholipid antibodies [13–16]. Antiphospholipid antibodies, β_2GPI-dependent aCL, and antiprothrombin, have been associated with cardiovascular disease (myocardial infarction, stroke, carotid stenosis) [12,17]. Anti-β_2GPI antibodies have been reported as more specific for thrombosis and APS than aCL antibodies [18], and recent prospective studies have shown that aCL antibodies, particularly β_2GPI-dependent, or anti-β_2GPI antibodies are important predictors for arterial thrombosis (myocardial infarction and stroke) in men [12,17,19].

Some aCL antibodies obtained from patients with APS crossreacted with oxLDL [40], providing initial direct clues that antiphospholipid antibodies participate in atherosclerosis. β_2GPI was found in human and rabitt atherosclerotic lesions with oxLDL, immunoreactive CD4/CD8 lymphocytes and immunoglobulins [20,21]. These findings provide additional support to the hypothesis that β_2GPI and anti-β_2GPI antibodies play a pathogenic role in the development of thrombosis, particularly arterial thrombosis (atherosclerosis) in SLE and APS patients. The development of larger fatty streaks in mice that received syngeneic lymphocytes from β_2GPI-immunized LDL-receptor deficient mice compared with control mice that received lymphocytes from mice immunized with bovine albumin [41]. This murine experimental model provided direct evidence that antigen β_2GPI-reactive T cells promote atherogenesis.

Immunologic mechanisms of atherosclerosis

Atherosclerosis is a multifactorial pathologic process in which arteries undergo thickening of the intima and smooth muscle layer causing a decrease in their elasticity. The blood vessels commonly affected by this process include the aorta, coronary, and cerebral arteries. The appearance of lipid laden foam cells in the arterial intima is a characteristic hystologic finding of early atherosclerotic lesions. Increased cholesterol blood levels are commonly associated with increased LDL. The combination of high [7] LDL with arterial shear stress may produce vascular inflammation that promotes the adherence of circulating monocytes to endothelial cells and the migration of these elements (LDL and monocytes) into the intima. Oxidatively-modified LDL (oxLDL) from vascular inflammation (and oxidative stress) further activates and attracts inflammatory cells to the site of the arterial lesion. The activation of macrophages would set off a series of pro-inflammatory events that include the expression of surface receptors, the intracellular influx of LDL, and the foam cell formation (oxLDL-loaded macrophages). Diverse pro-inflammatory or adhesion molecules also participate in atherogenesis. These molecules participate under complicated inter-related conditions and include: monocyte chemo-attractant protein-1 (MCP-1), macrophage colony-stimulating factor, interferon-γ, tumor necrosis factor-α (TNF-α), interleukine-4 (IL-4), platelet-derived growth factor, heparin-binding EGF-like growth factor, intercellular adhesion molecules, vascular cell adhesion molecules, endothelial selectin, and so on [42–45]. In addition, macrophage scavenger receptors and various cell–cell interactions, possibly via CD40 and CD40 ligands, have been reported to be involved in the development of atheroma [46].

It is widely accepted that LDL must be modified before is taken up by macrophages via scavenger receptors, and oxidation of LDL represents one such mechanism [27]. Normal blood levels of native (unmodified) LDL and perhaps, minimally modified LDL, are maintained by an LDL receptor uptake mechanism on endothelial and monocyte/macrophage cells. LDL receptors are downregulated to prevent excessive intracellular lipid accumulation. OxLDL is removed at a higher rate by macrophage scavenger receptors that are not downregulated, making possible an excessive intracellular accumulation of oxLDL and foam cell formation. When the endothelial surface of the atherosclerotic lesion becomes damaged and unstable, it may rupture into the arterial lumen. This event is followed by the activation of blood coagulation mechanisms such as platelet aggregation and thrombi formation, which can result in a complete occlusion of the blood vessel and tissue or organ necrosis, as seen in acute myocardial and cerebral infarction.

Oxidative modification of low-densitity lipoproetin

OxLDL plays a central pathogenic role in atherosclerosis [6]. The LDL particle contains phospholipids, free cholesterols, cholesteryl esters, triglycerides, and apolipoprotein B (apoB). Both the lipids and apoB lipoprotein are susceptible to oxidation, and apoB may break down into fragments of different sizes (from 14 kDa to over 550 kDa) by this process [47]. An important feature of LDL's oxidation is the breakdown of polyunsaturated fatty acids into a broad array of smaller fragments (ie, aldehydes and ketones bodies) that may conjugate to amino lipids or to apoB [48]. The polyunsaturated fatty acids in cholesterol esters, phospholipids, and triglycerides are also affected by free radical-initiated oxidation and can participate in a chain of reactions that further amplify the damage.

Recently, two significant oxidized fatty acid components have been described, 9- or 13-hydroxyoctadecadienoic acid (9-HODE and 13-HODE). These oxidized fatty acids activate peroxisome proliferator-activator receptor γ (PPARγ), a transcriptional regulator of genes linked to lipid metabolism that upregulate the CD36 scavenger receptor [49]. Thus, lipid components of oxLDL generated by activation of PPARγ can promote foam cell formation.

Linoleic acid is a predominant polyunsaturated fatty acid in LDL present mainly as cholesterol ester [50]. In mildly oxidized LDL, cholesteryl hydroperoxyoctadecadienoic acid (chol-HPODE) and cholesteryl hydroxyoctadecadienoic acid are the main products of oxidation. [51] It has been reported that chol-HPODE inactivates platelet-derived growth factor [52]. The oxidative breakdown of either free polyunsaturated fatty acids or those esterified at the sn-2 position of phospholipids may result in fatty acid hydroperoxides.

The fatty acid hydroperoxides formed may produce highly reactive products containing aldehyde and ketone functions. Such active functions can form Schiff base adducts with lysine residues of the apoB moiety of LDL. Cholesterol is also converted to oxysterols and it is especially oxidized at the seven position. 7-Hydroxycholesterol (both free and esterified) is the major oxysterol formed during early events in LDL oxidation, with 7-ketocholesterol dominating at later stages [53]. Recent studies have indicated that elevated plasma level of 7β-hydroxycholesterol is associated with an increased risk of atherosclerosis [54]. As a result of oxidation, a large number of oxidative structures are literally generated.

Chemically modified LDLs, such as MDA-LDL, acetylated-LDL and Cu^{2+}-oxLDL, have been extensively used to study atherogenic mechanisms. Small amounts of Cu^{2+} can induce LDL oxidation, resulting in highly reproducible LDL damage [55]. This process leads to an oxidized LDL structure that shares many functional properties with the LDL oxidized by cells or to oxLDL extracted from arterial atherosclerotic plaques. Incubation of LDL with several different types of cells, or with Cu^{2+} even in the absence of cells, results in an oxLDL structure with similar properties [56]. There is general consensus that Cu^{2+}-oxidized LDL is a relevant autoantigen because the oxLDL found in atheromatous lesions and the oxLDL extracted from atherosclerotic lesions exhibited similar physicochemical and immunologic properties to the Cu^{2+}-oxLDL [21]. Thus, Cu^{2+}-mediated oxLDL seems to be a more suitable model for physiologic LDL rather than other chemically modified LDL, such as MDA-LDL.

Regulation of low-density lipoprotein oxidation

Generalized immunologic vascular (endothelial) injury as seen in patients with autoimmune diseases may affect natural antioxidant mechanisms, making possible the oxidation of LDL. Ongoing lipid peroxidation (oxidative stress) has been demonstrated in patients with rheumatic diseases and vascular involvement [57], including patients with the antiphospholipid syndrome [58]. The presence of oxidative stress was assessed by different methods: urinary excretion of arachidonic acid metabolites (isoprostanes F2α), which is a marker in vivo of lipid peroxidation, chemiluminescence using a monocloanal antibody E06 specific for oxidized phopholipids, and multiple serum markers of protein oxidation by ELISA, acid hydrolysis and high-performance liquid chromatography.

The high-density lipoprotein (HDL)-associated enzyme paraoxonase 1 (PON1) has antioxidant activity that protects LDL from oxidation [59]. Decreased PON1 activity has been shown in patients with high serum levels of aCL antibodies [60]. Furthermore, IgG anti-β_2GPI antibodies have been associated with reduced PON1 activity in patients with SLE and primary APS [61]. PON1 activity is also known to increase with lipid-lowering drugs [62], and in one study, cholesterol-lowering statins prevented the in vitro endothelial cell activation induced by anti-β_2GPI antibodies [63]. Antioxidant treatment for 4 to 6 weeks has been observed to decrease the titer of circulating aCL antibodies in patients with SLE and APS [64].

In addition to PON1, other lipid oxidation mechanisms operating in autoimmune diseases have been investigated. Increased activity of vasoactive isoprostanes ($F_{2\alpha}$-III and $F_{2\alpha}$-VI) has been reported in these patients indicating in vivo oxidative stress, likely resulting in oxLDL formation [65]. Also, increased hydrolytic activity of phospholipase A2 and platelet-activating factor acetylhydrolase (PAF-AH) (Lp-PLA2) damaging LDL phospholipids may be responsible for the generation of pro-inflammatory molecules, possibly perpetuating a cycle of inflammation and oxidation of LDL [66].

Macrophages: role of scavenger and Fcγ receptors

Macrophages receptors for LDL were first described by Goldstein and Brown [67,68]. Theses receptors are downregulated to prevent lipid overloading. Another type of chemically modified-LDL macrophage receptors was later described and named scavenger receptors [67,69]. These scavenger receptors are not downregulated and chronic or excessive exposure to modified LDL may lead to the accumulation of massive amounts of intracellular lipids in macrophages, a process that may result in the formation of macrophage-derived lipid laden foam cells. Initially, acetylated-LDL was used to study scavenger receptors, but acetylation was not seen under physiologic conditions. In contrast, Cu^{2+} or Fe^{2+} oxLDL was described as a more physiologic ligand for scavenger receptors. Scavenger receptors (ie, SR-A) were first cloned by Kodama and colleagues [70,71], and shown to be specific for both acetylated-LDL and Cu^{2+}-oxLDL. This was followed by the description of several different types of scavenger receptors, that is, MARCO (a novel macrophage receptor with collagenous structure), SR-B1, CD36, Macrosialin, CD68, LOX-1, SREC, SRPSOX, and so on [72–79].

The in vitro macrophage uptake of ^{125}I-Cu^{2+}-oxLDL was significantly enhanced in the presence of β$_2$GPI and IgG anti-β$_2$GPI autoantibodies [23]. Similarly, the macrophage uptake of liposomes containing β$_2$GPI ligands (oxLig-1 and oxLig-2) was also enhanced, confirming the previous results [22,24,25] These findings indicated that IgG anti-β$_2$GPI autoantibodies may be pro-atherogenic. The in vivo oxLDL uptake is likely mediated by macrophage Fcγ receptors rather than by scavenger receptors. In contrast, Fcμ receptors have poor phagocytic properties, possibly making IgM class of autoantibodies or natural antibodies anti-atherogenic (or protective).

Role of oxidative low-density lipoprotein/β$_2$-glycoprotein I complexes in atherogenesis

β$_2$GPI is a 50-kDa single-chain polypeptide composed of 326 amino acid residues, arranged in five homologous repeats known as complement control protein domains. β$_2$GPI's fifth domain contains a patch of positively charged amino acids that likely represents the binding region for phospholipids [80,81]. β$_2$GPI binds strongly to negatively charged molecules, such as phospholipids, heparin, and certain lipoproteins as well as to activated platelets and apoptotic cell membranes. This binding may aid the clearance of apototic cells from circulation [82]. Further, β$_2$GPI may have anticoagulant properties, as it has been shown to inhibit the intrinsic coagulation pathway, prothrombinase activity, and adenosine diphosphate (ADP)-dependent platelet aggregation [83]. It has also been reported to interact with several components of the protein C, protein S anticoagulant system [84].

We recently demonstrated the specific interaction between Cu^{2+}-oxLDL and β$_2$GPI by ELISA [22–25]. Thus, oxLDL but not native LDL, binds β$_2$GPI and anti-β$_2$GPI autoantibodies. Two chloroform-extractable lipids (oxLig-1 and oxLig-2) were identified as the LDL-derived ligands for the specific interaction between oxLDL and β$_2$GPI. These oxLDL-derived β$_2$GPI ligands were further purified by reverse-phase HPLC and their structures were identified as 7-ketocholesteryl-9-carboxynonanoate [9-oxo-9-(7-ketocholest-5-en-3-yloxy) nonanoic acid] and 7-ketocholesteryl-12-carboxy (keto) dodecanoate, respectively. Cholesteryl linoleate present in LDL is a major core lipid, and represents the most probable candidate for a precursor of these ligands. The initial in vitro interaction of Cu^{2+}-oxLDL with β$_2$GPI is due to electrostatic interactions between ω-carboxyl functions and lysine residues of β$_2$GPI and is reversible by Mg^{2+} treatment. This interaction later progresses to a much more stable bond such as Schiff base formation with an ω-aldehyde. Interestingly, the negative charges generated by Cu^{2+}-oxLDL were neutralized by the interaction with β$_2$GPI. These complexes have been demonstrated in some patients with SLE and APS

[22]. The strength of the bond formed and the neutralization of the charges by the complexes may contribute to their stability in the blood stream.

Pro-atherogenic role of oxidative low-density lipoprotein/β₂-glycoprotein I complexes

Lipid peroxidation and oxLDL production are common in patients with some systemic autoimmune diseases [57,85,86]. oxLDL, not native LDL, binds β_2GPI in vitro, initially forming dissociable electrostatic complexes followed by more stable complexes bound by covalent interactions. Circulating oxLDL/β_2GPI complexes have been detected in some autoimmune diseases [27,87]. High serum levels of stable oxLDL/β_2GPI complexes were detected by ELISA in 70% to 80% of patients with SLE and systemic sclerosis (SSc). Patients with rheumatoid arthritis (RA) showed a slight increase of oxLDL/β_2GPI complexes compared to healthy controls. Unlike RA, both SLE and SSc are characterized by widespread vascular abnormalities. Serum levels of oxLDL/β_2GPI complexes were [13] also significantly elevated in patients to secondary APS and in SLE patients without APS compared to healthy controls. However, these complexes were not associated with SLE disease activity or any major clinical manifestation of APS [87]. Although it can be hypothesized that this interaction might be related to chronic vascular inflammation that occurs in autoimmune patients, the exact in vivo mechanism(s) that oxidizes LDL and forms oxLDL/β_2GPI complexes are not fully understood. It is possible that the interaction between β_2GPI and oxLDL minimizes the inflammatory properties of oxLDL while promoting its clearance from circulation. In addition, the binding of β_2GPI to oxLDL may likely occur inside the arterial wall, as the intima microenvironment is conducive to further inflammation, oxidation, cell activation, and macrophage uptake of oxLDL/β_2GPI complexes. Serum levels of oxLDL/β_2GPI complexes fluctuated widely when measured in samples obtained at different time intervals over a 12-month follow-up from [6] SLE patients. This suggests that oxidation and formation of complexes are very active processes under unknown regulatory mechanism(s). Stable oxLDL/β_2GPI complexes may be clinically relevant, as they have been implicated as atherogenic autoantigens, and their presence may represent a risk factor or an indirect but significant contributor for thrombosis and atherosclerosis in patients with an autoimmune background.

Autoantibodies to oxidative low-density lipoprotein/β₂-glycoprotein I complexes in autoimmune-mediated atherosclerosis

OxLDL/β_2GPI complexes are immunogenic. Serum levels of IgG anti-oxLDL/β_2GPI antibodies were measured in the same group of SLE, SSc, and RA patients. SLE and SSc patients had significantly higher levels of anti-oxLDL/β_2GPI antibodies compared to the controls. RA patients showed higher antibody levels than the controls, but this difference was not statistically significant. The association of IgG anti-oxLDL/β_2GPI antibodies with the major clinical manifestations of APS was evaluated [27,88–90]. There was a stronger correlation with arterial thrombosis compared to venous thrombosis and pregnancy morbidity. Further, the positive predictive value of IgG anti-oxLDL/β_2GPI antibodies for [14] total thrombosis (arterial and venous) in patients with secondary APS was 92%, and for arterial thrombosis was 88.9%. In contrast, the positive predictive value for venous thrombosis was not statistically significant at 77.7%. In addition, anti-oxLDL/β_2GPI antibodies were present in three of four SLE patients with active disease followed over a 12-month period, while two patients with inactive disease and oxLDL/β_2GPI complexes did not have these antibodies [87].

The coexistence of oxLDL/β_2GPI autoantibodies with oxLDL/β_2GPI complexes suggest that these two elements interact perhaps forming circulating immune complexes (oxLDL/β_2GPI/antibody). Such immune complexes have been recently detected in patients with SLE or APS [22]. These observations, along with the increased in vitro uptake of oxLDL/β_2GPI complexes by macrophage in the presence of anti-oxLDL/β_2GPI antibodies [23–25], provide an explanation for the accelerated (premature) development of atherosclerosis in autoimmune patients. Although preliminary, IgG anti-oxLDL/β_2GPI antibodies represent a distinct subset of antiphospholipid antibodies (ie, anti-β_2GPI) that coexist with other antiphospholipid antibodies. Thus, IgG anti-oxLDL/β_2GPI antibodies appear to be useful serologic markers for atherosclerotic risk in autoimmune patients with high specificity for APS.

Summary and clinical significance

The binding of oxLDL with β_2GPI to form circulating complexes strongly suggests that these complexes are atherogenic autoantigens. The nature of the binding has been further characterized, and the oxLDL-derived ligand (oxLig-1) specific for β_2GPI has been identified and synthesized. SLE and APS patients produce autoantibodies to this complex, and the resulting circulating immune complexes may accelerate the development of atherosclerosis. The physiologic relevance of these findings has been demonstrated in vitro by the enhanced macrophage uptake of oxLDL/β_2GPI/antibody complexes. The participation of macrophage Fcγ receptors in the uptake of oxLDL-containing complexes [15] seems to be particularly important to explain the development of foam cells and autoimmune-mediated atherosclerotic plaques.

Are there other molecules, antigens, antibodies, or other interactions playing a role in the development of atherosclerosis? OxLDL is highly pro-inflammatory and immunogenic, making this molecule a prime target for natural defense mechanisms. The resulting complexes may not be irreversibly harmful if the process is self-limiting or self-contained.

Chronic and more severe inflammatory processes, especially in autoimmune prone individuals, may induce immune responses that perpetuate a pathologic process, that is, atherosclerosis. C-reactive protein (CRP), fibrinogen, (TNF-α), heat-shock protein, homocysteine, and so on, are being used to assess the risk of cardiovascular disease. However, the exact mode of action of these molecules is not completely understood. It has been recently described that oxLDL can interact with CRP to form pro-atherogenic complexes. The product of these and other interactions may not only cause vascular inflammation but also trigger autoantibodies and immune complexes that accelerate the development of atherosclerosis.

The development of ELISA test kits to measure oxLDL/β_2GPI complexes and anti-oxLDL/β_2GPI antibodies had provided additional tools to further study the role of the humoral immune response in the atherosclerotic process. Stable and likely pathogenic oxLDL/β_2GPI complexes were demonstrated in the serum of SLE, SSc, and APS patients. Anti-oxLDL/β_2GPI antibodies were detected in SLE and SSc patients, both diseases characterized by generalized vascular complications. Further, the association of these antibodies with arterial thrombosis was stronger than venous thrombosis in APS patients. The role of oxLDL/β_2GPI complexes and autoantibodies to these complexes in the vascular complications of SSc remain to be further studied. At this point, these results should be interpreted in the context of an autoimmune disease. However, oxLDL/β_2GPI complexes have been demonstrated in patients with syphilis, infectious endocarditis, type 2 diabetes mellitus, and chronic nephritis, indicating that oxidation of LDL and the formation of complexes with β_2GPI is not restricted to SLE. In contrast, none of these patients developed significant levels of anti-oxLDL/β_2GPI antibodies. These antibodies seem to be restricted to patients with SLE and APS. Thus, it can be hypothesized that these antibodies accelerate the development of atherosclerosis in autoimmune patients.

References

[1] Ward MM. Premature morbidity from cardiovascular and cerebrovascular diseases in women with systemic lupus erythematosus. Arthritis Rheum 1999;42:338–46.

[2] Aranow C, Ginzler EM. Epidemiology of cardiovascular disease in systemic lupus erythematosus. Lupus 2000;9:166–9.

[3] Schattner A, Liang MH. The cardiovascular burden of lupus; a complex challenge. Arch Intern Med 2003;163:1507–10.

[4] Steinbrecher UP, Parthasarathy S, Leake DS, et al. Modification of low-density lipoprotein by endothelial cells involves lipid peroxidation and degradation of low-density lipoprotein phospholipids. Proc Natl Acad Sci USA 1984;81:3883–7.

[5] Steinberg D, Parthasarathy S, Carew TE, et al. Beyond cholesterol. Modifications of low-density lipoprotein that increase its atherogenicity. N Engl J Med 1989;320:915–24.

[6] Steinberg D. Low-density lipoprotein oxidation and its pathobiological significance. J Biol Chem 1997;272:20963–6.

[7] Heinecke JW. Mechanisms of oxidative damage of low-density lipoprotein in human atherosclerosis. Curr Opin Lipid 1997;8:268–74.

[8] Hughes GRV, Harris EN, Gharavi AE. The anticardiolipin syndrome. J Rheumatol 1986; 13:486–9.

[9] Harris EN, Gharavi AE, Boey ML, et al. Anticardiolipin antibodies: detection by radioimmunoassay and association with thrombosis in systemic lupus erythematosus. Lancet 1983; 2:1211–4.

[10] Ginsburg KS, Liang MH, Newcomer L, et al. Anticardiolipin antibodies and the risk for ischemic stroke and venous thrombosis. Ann Intern Med 1992;117:997–1002.

[11] Roubey RA. Autoantibodies to phospholipid-binding plasma proteins: a new view of lupus anticoagulants and other "antiphospholipid" autoantibodies. Blood 1994;84: 2854–67.

[12] Vaarala O. Antiphospholipid antibodies in myocardial infarction. Lupus 1998;7:S132–4.

[13] McNeil HP, Simpson RJ, Chesterman CN, et al. Anti-phospholipid antibodies are directed against a complex antigen that includes a lipid-binding inhibitor of coagulation: β_2-glycoprotein I (apolipoprotein H). Proc Natl Acad Sci USA 1990;87:4120–4.

[14] Galli M, Comfurius P, Maassen C, et al. Anticardiolipin antibodies (ACA) directed not to cardiolipin but to a plasma protein cofactor. Lancet 1990;335:1544–7.

[15] Matsuura E, Igarashi Y, Fujimoto M, et al. Heterogeneity of anticardiolipin antibodies defined by the anticardiolipin cofactor. J Immunol 1992;148:3885–91.

[16] Matsuura E, Igarashi Y, Yasuda T, et al. Anticardiolipin antibodies recognize β_2-glycoprotein I structure altered by interacting with an oxygen modified solid phase surface. J Exp Med 1994;179:457–62.

[17] Brey RL, Abbott RD, Curb JD, et al. β_2-glycoprotein I dependent anticardiolipin antibodies and the risk of ischemic stroke and myocardial infarction. Stroke 2001;32:1701–6.

[18] Tsutsumi A, Matsuura E, Ichikawa K, et al. Antibodies to β_2-glycoprotein I and clinical manifestations in patients with systemic lupus erythematosus. Arthritis Rheum 1996;39: 1466–74.

[19] Lopez LR, Dier KJ, Lopez D, et al. Anti-β_2-glycoprotein I and antiphosphatidylserine antibodies are predictors of arterial thrombosis in patients with antiphospholipid syndrome. Am J Clin Pathol 2004;121:142–9.

[20] George J, Harats D, Gilburd B, et al. Immunolocalization of β_2-glycoprotein I (apolipoprotein H) to human atherosclerotic plaques: potential implications for lesion progression. Circulation 1999;99:2227–30.

[21] Yla-Herttuala S, Palinski W, Rosenfeld ME, et al. Evidence for presence of oxidatively modified lowdensity lipoprotein in atherosclerotic lesions of rabbit and man. J Clin Invest 1989; 85:1086–95.

[22] Kobayashi K, Kishi M, Atsumi T, et al. Circulating oxidized LDL forms complexes with 2-glycoprotein I: implication as an atherogenic autoantigen. J Lipid Res 2003;44:716–26.

[23] Hasunuma Y, Matsuura E, Makita Z, et al. Involvement of β_2-glycoprotein I and anticardiolipin antibodies in oxidatively modified low-density lipoprotein uptake by macrophages. Clin Exp Immunol 1997;107:569–73.

[24] Kobayashi K, Matsuura E, Liu Q, et al. A specific ligand for β_2-19 glycoprotein I mediates autoantibody-dependent uptake of oxidized low density lipoprotein by macrophages. J Lipid Res 2001;42:697–709.

[25] Liu Q, Kobayashi K, Inagaki J, et al. ω-carboxyl variants of 7-ketocholesteryl esters are ligands for β_2-glycoprotein I and mediate antibody-dependent uptake of oxidized LDL by macrophages. J Lipid Res 2002;43:1486–95.

[26] American Heart Association. Heart disease and stroke statistics—2005 update. www.americanheart.org.

[27] Ross R. Atherosclerosis: an inflammatory disease. N Engl J Med 1999;340:115–26.

[28] Steinberg D. Atherogenesis in perspective: hypercholesterolemia and inflammation as partners in crime. Nat Med 2002;8:1211–7.

[29] Berliner JA, Heinecke JW. The role of oxidized lipoproteins in atherogenesis. Free Radic Biol Med 1996;20:707–27.

[30] McMurray HF, Parthasarathy S, Steinberg D. Oxidatively modified lowdensity lipoprotein is a chemoattractant for human T lymphocytes. J Clin Invest 1993;92:1004–8.

[31] Virella G, Atchley DH, Koskinen S, et al. Proatherogenic and pro-inflammatory properties of immune complexes prepared with purified human oxLDL antibodies and human oxLDL. Clin Immunol 2002;105:81–92.

[32] Salonen JT, Yla-Herttuala S, Yamamoto R, et al. Autoantibodies against oxidized LDL and progression of carotid atherosclerosis. Lancet 1992;339:883–7.

[33] Esdaile JM, Abrahamowicz M, Grodzicky T, et al. Traditional Framingham risk factors fail to fully account for accelerated atherosclerosis in systemic lupus erythematosus. Arthritis Rheum 2001;44:2331–7.

[34] Petri M. Autoimmune thrombosis. In: Asherson RA, Cervera R, Piette J, Schoenfeld Y, editors. The antiphospholipid syndrome. Amsterdam: Elsevier Science; 2002. p. 11–20.

[35] Thomas RH. Hypercoagulability syndromes. Arch Intern Med 2001;161:2433–9.

[36] Wahl DG, Guillemin F, de Maistre E, et al. Risk for venous thrombosis related to anti-phospholipid antibodies in systemic lupus erythematosus: a meta analysis. Lupus 1997;6: 467–73.

[37] Shah NM, Khamashta MA, Atsumi T, et al. Outcome of patients with anticardiolipin anti-bodies: a 10 year follow-up of 52 patients. Lupus 1998;7:3–6.

[38] Khamashta MA, Cuadrado MJ, Mujic F, et al. The management of thrombosis in the anti-phospholipid-antibody syndrome. N Engl J Med 1995;332:993–7.

[39] Cervera R, Piette JC, Font J, et al, and the Euro-Phospholipid Project Group. Antiphospho-lipid syndrome. Clinical and immunologic manifestations and patterns of disease expression in a cohort of 1,000 patients. Arthritis Rheum 2002;46:1019–27.

[40] Vaarala O, Alfthan G, Jauhiainen M, et al. Crossreaction between antibodies to oxidised low-density lipoprotein and to cardiolipin in systemic lupus erythematosus. Lancet 1993; 341:923–5.

[41] George J, Harats D, Gilburd B, et al. Adoptive transfer of β_2-glycoprotein I-reactive lym-phocytes enhances early atherosclerosis in LDL receptor-deficient mice. Circulation 2000; 102:1822–7.

[42] Cushing SD, Berliner JA, Valente AJ, et al. Minimally modified low-density lipoprotein induces monocyte chemotactic protein 1 in human endothelial cells and smooth muscle cells. Proc Natl Acad Sci USA 1990;87:5134–8.

[43] Rajavashisth TB, Andalibi A, Territo MC, et al. Induction of endothelial cell expression of granulocyte and macrophage colony-stimulating factors by modified low-density lipopro-teins. Nature 1990;344:254–7.

[44] Nakata A, Miyagawa J, Yamashita S, et al. Localization of heparin-binding epidermal growth factor-like growth factor in human coronary arteries. Possible roles of HBEGF in the formation of coronary atherosclerosis. Circulation 1996;94:2778–86.

[45] Frostegard J, Wu R, Haegerstrand A, et al. Mononuclear leukocytes exposed to oxidized low density lipoprotein secrete a factor that stimulates endothelial cells to express adhesion mol-ecules. Atherosclerosis 1993;103:213–9.

[46] Mach F, Schonbeck U, Sukhova GK, et al. Reduction of atherosclerosis in mice by inhibi-tion of CD40 signalling. Nature 1998;394:200–3.

[47] Fong LG, Parthasarathy S, Witztum JL, et al. Nonenzymatic oxidative cleavage of peptide bonds in apoprotein B-100. J Lipid Res 1987;28:1466–77.

[48] Esterbauer H, Jurgens G, Quehenberger O, et al. Autoxidation of human low density lipo-protein: loss of polyunsaturated fatty acids and vitamin E and generation of aldehydes. J Lipid Res 1987;28:495–509.

[49] Nagy L, Tontonoz P, Alvarez JG, et al. Oxidized LDL regulates macrophage gene expression through ligand activation of PPAR. Cell 1998;93:229–40.

[50] Weidtmann A, Scheithe R, Hrboticky N, et al. Mildly oxidized LDL induces platelet aggre-gation through activation of phsopholipase A2. Arterioscler Thromb Vasc Biol 1995;15: 1131–8.

[51] Kritharides L, Jessup W, Gifford J, et al. A method for defining the stages of low density lipoprotein oxidation by the separation of cholesterol and cholesteryl ester-oxidation products using HPLC. Anal Biochem 1993;213:79–89.

[52] van Heek M, Schmitt D, Toren P, et al. Cholesteryl hydroperoxyoctadecadienoate from oxidized low-density lipoprotein inactivated platelet-derived growth factor. J Biol Chem 1998; 273:19405–10.

[53] Brown AJ, Leong SL, Dean RT, et al. 7-Hydroperoxycholesterol and its products in oxidized low-density lipoprotein and human atherosclerotic plaque. J Lipid Res 1997;38: 1730–45.

[54] Brown AJ, Jessup W. Oxysterols and atherosclerosis. Atherosclerosis 1999;142:1–28.

[55] Kleinveld HA, Hak-Lemmers HLM, Stalenhoef AFH, et al. Improved measurement of low-density-lipoprotein susceptibility to copper-induced oxidation: application of a short procedure for isolating low-density lipoprotein. Clin Chem 1992;38:2066–72.

[56] Parthasarathy S, Fong LG, Quinn MT, et al. Oxidative modification of LDL: comparison between cell-mediated and copper-mediated modification. Eur Heart J 1990;11(Suppl.):83–7.

[57] Ames PRJ, Alves J, Murat I, et al. Oxidative stress in systemic lupus erythematosus and allied conditions with vascular involvement. Rheumatol 1999;38:529–34.

[58] Ames PRJ, Tommasino C, Alves J, et al. Antioxidant susceptibility of pathogenic pathways in subjects with antiphospholipid antibodies: a pilot study. Lupus 2000;9:688–95.

[59] Durrington PN, Mackness B, Mackness MI. Paraoxonase and atherosclerosis. Arterioscler Thromb Vasc Biol 2001;21:473–80.

[60] Lambert M, Boullier A, Hachulla E, et al. Paraoxonase activity is dramatically decreased in patients positive for anticardiolipin antibodies. Lupus 2000;9:299–300.

[61] Delgado Alves J, Ames PR, Donohue S, et al. Antibodies to high-density lipoprotein and β_2-glycoprotein I are inversely correlated with Paraoxonase activity in Systemic lupus erythematosus and primary antiphospholipid syndrome. Arthritis Rheum 2002;46:2686–94.

[62] Belogh Z, Seres I, Harangi M, et al. Gemfibrozil increases paraoxonase activity in type β_2 diabetic patients: a new hypothesis of the beneficial action of fibrates? Diabetes Metab 2001;27:604–10.

[63] Meroni PL, Raschi E, Testoni C, et al. Statins prevent endothelial cell activation induced by antiphospholipid (anti-β_2-glycoprotein I) antibodies. Effect on the proadhesive and proinflammatory phenotype. Arthritis Rheum 2001;44:2870–8.

[64] Ferro D, Iuliano L, Violi F, et al. Antioxidant treatment decreases the titer of circulating anticardiolipin antibodies. Arthritis Rheum 2002;46:3110–2.

[65] Pratico D, Ferro D, Iuliano L, et al. Ongoing prothrombotic state in patients with antiphospholipid antibodies: a role for increased lipid peroxidation. Blood 1999;93:3401–7.

[66] Hurt-Camejo E, Paredes S, Masana L, et al. Elevated levels of small, low-density lipoprotein with high affinity for arterial matrix components in patients with rheumatoid arthritis. Possible contribution of phospholipase A2 to this atherogenic profile. Arthritis Rheum 2001;44: 2761–7.

[67] Goldstein JL, Ho YK, Basu SK, et al. Binding site on macrophages that mediates uptake and degradation of acetylated low-density lipoprotein, producing massive cholesterol deposition. Proc Natl Acad Sci USA 1979;76:333–7.

[68] Yamamoto T, Davis CG, Brown MS, et al. The human LDL receptor: a cysteine-rich protein with multiple Alu sequences in its mRNA. Cell 1984;39:27–38.

[69] Brown MS, Goldstein JL. Scavenger cell receptor shared. Nature 1985;316:680–1.

[70] Kodama T, Reddy P, Kishimoto C, et al. Purification and characterization of a bovine acetyl low-density lipoprotein receptor. Proc Natl Acad Sci USA 1988;85:9238–42.

[71] Kodama T, Freeman M, Rohrer L, et al. Type I macrophage scavenger receptor contains alpha-helical and collagen-like coiled coils. Nature 1990;343:531–5.

[72] Elomaa O, Kangas M, Sahlberg C, et al. Cloning of a novel bacteria-binding receptor structurally related to scavenger receptors and expressed in a subset of macrophages. Cell 1995;80: 603–9.

[73] Elomaa O, Sankala M, Pikkarainen T, et al. Structure of the human macrophage MARCO receptor and characterization of its bacteria-binding region. J Biol Chem 1998;273: 4530–8.

[74] Ramprasad MP, Fischer W, Witztum JL, et al. The 94- to 97-kDa mouse macrophage membrane protein that recognizes oxidized low density lipoprotein and phosphatidylserine-rich liposomes is identical to macrosialin, the mouse homologue of human CD68. Proc Natl Acad Sci USA 1995;92:9580–4.

[75] Sambrano GR, Steinberg D. Recognition of oxidatively damaged and apoptotic cells by an oxidized low density lipoprotein receptor on mouse peritoneal macrophages: role of membrane phosphatidylserine. Proc Natl Acad Sci USA 1995;92:1396–400.

[76] Rigotti A, Acton SL, Krieger M. The class B scavenger receptors SR-BI and CD36 are receptors for anionic phospholipids. J Biol Chem 1995;270:16221–4.

[77] Sawamura T, Kume N, Aoyama T, et al. An endothelial receptor for oxidized low-density lipoprotein. Nature 1997;386:73–7.

[78] Minami M, Kume N, Shimaoka T, et al. Expression of SR-PSOX, a novel cell-surface scavenger receptor for phosphatidylserine and oxidized LDL in human atherosclerotic lesions. Arterioscler Thromb Vasc Biol 2001;21:1796–800.

[79] Shimaoka T, Kume N, Minami M, et al. Molecular cloning of a novel scavenger receptor for oxidized low-density lipoprotein, SR-PSOX, on macrophages. J Biol Chem 2000;275: 40663–6.

[80] Bouma B, de Groot PG, van den Elsen JM, et al. Adhesion mechanism of human β_2-glycoprotein I to phospholipids based on its crystal structure. EMBO J 1999;18:5166–74.

[81] Hoshino M, Hagihara Y, Nishii I, et al. Identification of the phospholipid-binding site of human β_2-glycoprotein I domain V by heteronuclear magnetic resonance. J Mol Biol 2000;304: 927–39.

[82] Inanc M, Radway-Bright EL, Isenberg DA. β_2-glycoprotein I and anti-β_2-glycoprotein I antibodies: where are we now? Br J Rheumatol 1997;36:1247–57.

[83] Sheng Y, Kandiah DA, Krilis SA. β_2-glycoprotein I: Target antigen for "antiphospholipid" antibodies. Immunological and molecular aspects. Lupus 1998;7:S5–9.

[84] Merrill JT, Zhang HW, Shen C, et al. Enhancement of Protein S anticoagulant function by β_2-glycoprotein I, a major target antigen of antiphospholipid antibodies: β_2-glycoprotein I interferes with binding of Protein S to its plasma inhibitor, C4b-binding protein. Thromb Haemost 1999;81:748–57.

[85] Morgan PE, Sturgess AD, Davies M. Increased levels of serum protein oxidation and correlation with disease activity in patients with systemic lupus erythematosus. Arthritis Rheum 2005;52:2069–79.

[86] Frostegard J, Svenungsson E, Wu R, et al. Lipid peroxidation is enhanced in patients with systemic lupus erythematosus and is associated with arterial and renal disease manifestations. Arthritis Rheum 2005;52:192–200.

[87] Lopez D, Garcia-Valladares I, Palafox-Sanchez C, et al. Oxidized low-density lipoprotein/β_2-glycoprotein I complexes and autoantibodies to oxLig-1/β_2-glycoprotein I in patients with systemic lupus erythematosus and antiphospholipid syndrome. Am J Clin Pathol 2004;121:426–36.

[88] Matsuura E, Kobayashi K, Inoue K, et al. Oxidized LDL/β_2-glycoprotein I complexes: new aspects in atherosclerosis. Lupus 2005;14:736–41.

[89] Lopez LR, Simpson DF, Hurley BL, et al. OxLDL/β_2-GPI complexes and autoantibodies in patients with systemic lupus erythematosus, systemic sclerosis and antiphospholipid syndrome. Pathogenic implications for vascular involvement. Ann N Y Acad Sci 2005;1051: 313–22.

[90] Lopez D, Kobayashi K, Merrill JT, et al. IgG Autoantibodies against β_2-glycoprotein I complexed with a lipid ligand derived from oxidized low-density lipoprotein are associated with arterial thrombosis in antiphospholipid syndrome. Clin Dev Immunol 2003;10: 203–11.

ELSEVIER
SAUNDERS

Rheum Dis Clin N Am
32 (2006) 553–573

RHEUMATIC
DISEASE CLINICS
OF NORTH AMERICA

Pediatric Antiphospholipid Syndrome

Rolando Cimaz, MD[a],*, Elodie Descloux[b]

[a]Département de Pédiatrie, pavillon S, Hopital Edouard Herriot, and Université Claude
Bernard- Lyon 1, 5 Place d'Arsonval 69437, Lyon, France
[b]Service de médecine interne-pathologie vasculaire, unité Giraud Sud, pavillon 1K Centre
Hospitalier Lyon Sud 69495, Pierre-Benite cedex, France

Similar as in adults, antiphospholipid antibodies (aPL) have been recognized in a number of childhood conditions including pediatric autoimmune diseases, various infections, as well as in a small percentage of apparently healthy children [1–7]. Pathogenic mechanisms involved in pediatric antiphospholipid syndrome (APS) have not been thoroughly investigated, but it is generally assumed that they are similar to adults. However, there clearly are differences in the frequency of specific clinical events, because children do not have risk profiles that could be predisposing factors for thrombosis (eg, atherosclerosis, cigarette smoking, contraceptive medications).

Most of the clinical features that can occur in adults with aPL have also been described in children, but often just as individual case reports or small case series from single institutions. Large cohorts or multicenter studies on APS in pediatric population are rare, and consequently, there is very little accurate information on the pediatric aspects of APS. The aim of this review is to highlight relevant clinical advances in the field of pediatric APS.

Antiphospholipid antibodies in healthy children

aPL can be found in apparently healthy children; such naturally occurring aPL are usually present in low titer and could be the result of previous infections or vaccinations, common events in the pediatric populations [8–10].

A number of studies have addressed the frequency of anticardiolipin antibodies (aCL) in healthy children, but the findings are controversial, with prevalence figures ranging from 2% to 82% [9,11–16]. These discrepancies might be secondary to methodologic issues such as differences in inclusion

---

* Corresponding author.
  E-mail address: Roland.Cimaz@chu-lyon.fr (R. Cimaz).

criteria, cutoff values, and assay methods. Kontiainen and colleagues [14] tested aCL in 173 children with minor surgical or psychosomatic problems and found surprisingly high frequency of positive aCL (82%). A group of children with functional disorders was also studied by Rapizzi and colleagues [9], who found positive aCL in 28% of them. In contrast, five smaller studies have reported quite low frequencies of aCL (under 5%) in healthy children [11–13,15,16].

In a well-defined group of 61 apparently healthy children at regular preventive visits, a positivity of aCL in 11% and of anti-β2 glycoprotein I (anti-β$_2$GPI) in 7% of subjects was found, respectively [10]. Mean values of IgG and IgM aCL were comparable between different age groups, while the mean value of IgA aCL was significantly higher in blood donors than in preschool children and adolescents. Moreover, it was found that the mean value of IgG anti-β$_2$GPI was highest in preschool children, and in this group it was significantly higher than in adolescents and blood donors. It is possible that early ingestion of bovine β$_2$GPI found in milk and other nutritional products could act as an oral immunization agent and induce transient production of anti-β$_2$GPI in infants.

Lupus anticoagulants (LA) have also been described in healthy children [8, 7–19]. This is quite a common problem, because LA are often discovered incidentally in preoperative evaluations of children scheduled for adenotonsillectomy who present with prolonged activated partial thromboplastin time (aPTT). In many cases no definite diagnosis can be found, and the aPTT spontaneously corrects to the normal range [8]. Positive LA were identified in 7% of 61 apparently healthy children [7], and, similar to previous studies [8,17,18], no correlations between LA and aCL/anti-β$_2$GPI were observed.

Studies of children with aPL that have included healthy controls are summarized in Table 1.

Primary antiphospholipid syndrome

Primary APS (PAPS) in pediatric populations is very rare. The most frequently described types of thrombotic events were deep venous thrombosis

Table 1
Incidence of antiphospholipid antibodies in healthy children

Reference	Patients No.	% +aPL
Caporali 1991 [11]	42	IgG 0%; IgM 5%
Kontiainen 1996 [14]	173	IgG 82%
Singer 1997 [20]	20	IgG 10%
Kratz 1998 [15]	20	IgG 0% ; IgM 5%
Rapizzi 2000 [9]	100	IgG 26%; IgM & A 1%
Avcin 2001 [10]	61	IgG 11%

in the lower extremities, pulmonary embolism, and thrombotic complications in the central nervous system.

Manco-Johnson and Nuss identified LA in 25% of 78 consecutive children who were diagnosed with thromboses in their institution [21]. Clinical manifestations included deep venous thrombosis (six), central nervous system manifestations (five), pulmonary embolism (four), distal deep venous thrombosis (two), central venous thrombosis (two), and proximal arterial thrombosis (one). Fourteen were diagnosed with PAPS [21]. Von Scheven and colleagues [22] reported on clinical characteristics of five patients with PAPS in childhood, who presented with digital ischemia, stroke, chorea, adrenal insufficiency, and pulmonary vaso-occlusive disease.

Deep vein thrombosis (DVT) is the most common venous thrombotic condition reported in children associated with PAPS. In some cases, pulmonary embolism has been also described [23]. Pulmonary hypertension related to microthromboembolic phenomenon is rare but reported in children with PAPS [22]. In one report, a child with PAPS developed portal vein thrombosis [24]. Addison's disease and hypoadrenalism are also known to be caused by infarction of the adrenal glands due to aPL; this has also been reported in children with PAPS [22]. Myocardial infarction at a young age should prompt the clinician to search for aPL, as there have been rare reports of this association in children [25].

Cerebral ischemic stroke is the most common neurologic event reported in association with aPL, and the most common arterial thrombotic condition. It has been suggested by some authors that a significant proportion of children who suffer from idiopathic stroke, at any age, have elevated aPL levels [26–28]. Two large series of idiopathic cerebral venous and sinovenous thrombosis in children also have identified aPL as an important risk factor [29,30]. In children with sinovenous thrombosis, the frequency of prothrombotic disorders is 12% to 50%, and the presence of aCL is the most common acquired disorder. There are other less common arterial thrombotic conditions reported in children with PAPS. Transverse myelitis, seen rarely in children with systemic lupus, appears to be a possible thrombotic complication of PAPS [31]. Renal thrombotic microangiopathy, a rare finding in adults with APS, has been also described in an adolescent with PAPS who presented with severe hypertension, renal impairment, and a history of Raynaud's phenomenon [32]. Optic neuropathy has been reported also in PAPS in childhood [33].

Additionally, it has to be underlined that consensus criteria for APS may not be appropriate for children, and may fail to recognize significant group of pediatric patients with PAPS [34]. In fact, thromboses are very rare in children, and recurrent fetal losses are obviously not a pediatric problem. Available data from clinical studies suggest that other clinical features such as migraine, chorea, epilepsy, thrombocytopenia, and hemolytic anemia might also be associated with pediatric APS.

The outcome of APS in children has not been thoroughly studied. Gattorno and colleagues [35] investigated the long-term outcome of 14 pediatric patients with primary APS. Nine boys and five girls between 3 and 13 years of age (median, 9 years) were followed for a median of 9 years. Clinical features were deep venous thrombosis (six), cerebral stroke (five), peripheral artery occlusion (two), and myocardial infarction (one). During follow-up, four patients had one or more recurrences of vascular thrombosis, two patients developed the criteria for full-blown systemic lupus erythematosus (SLE) [36], and one patient developed a lupus-like syndrome. The percentage of progression to SLE or lupus-like syndrome in this pediatric cohort (21.4%) was almost double than that found in adult patients with primary APS [37]. In the three patients who developed SLE or lupus-like syndrome, the features of the disease occurred soon after the presentation of APS (9–14 months for full-blown SLE, 6 months for lupus-like disease). These findings suggest that a proportion of children who present with features of PAPS can progress in a relatively short time to SLE.

Secondary antiphospholipid syndrome

Systemic lupus erythematosus

SLE is the autoimmune disease where aPL occurs in highest percentage [15,38–48], and APS in children more frequently occurs in association with SLE or lupus-like disease than in the isolated, primary form. An analysis of 12 reported series in children with SLE yields a global prevalence of 48% (257 of 532) for aCL and 23% (136 of 593) for LA (Table 2).

A variety of clinical features have been reported to be present in aPL-positive children with SLE, including arterial and venous thromboses, different

Table 2
Antiphospholipid antibodies in pediatric systemic lupus erythematosus (case series)

Reference	Patients	% aPL+	% aCL+	% LA+	% Thrombosis
Shergy et al. 1988 [38]	32	50	50	—	0
Montes de Oca et al. 1991 [39]	120	19	—	19	9
Molta et al. 1993 [40]	37	38	19	11	8
Ravelli et al. 1994 [41]	30	87	87	20	3
Gattorno et al. 1995 [13]	19	90	79	42	16
Seaman et al. 1995 [42]	29	65	66	62	24
Massengill et al. 1997 [43]	36	67	50	6	—
Berube et al. 1998 [44]	59	—	19	24	17
Gedalia et al. 1998 [45]	36	—	37	—	8
Von Scheven et al. 2002 [46]	57	67	53	23	5
Campos et al. 2003 [47]	57	35	33	7	14
Levy et al. 2003 [48]	149	—	39	16	9

neurologic manifestations, and autoimmune cytopenias. The presence of aPL was most strongly associated with thromboses, particularly in the presence of a positive LA [48,49]. Thromboembolic events reported in studies and case reports include DVT, pulmonary embolism, superior vena cava thrombosis, ischemic stoke, retinal artery occlusion, renal artery occlusion, and transverse myelitis [38–40,47,50–53]. We have also seen such complications: Fig. 1 shows a thrombosis of the superior longitudinal sinus in a boy affected by APS secondary to SLE. This boy had onset of his disease at age 9, suffered from a DVT after 1 year, and at age 18 presented acute neurologic involvement with headache, paresthesia, drowsiness, and visual disturbances.

A recent study [54] has determined the association of aPL subtypes with thrombotic events (TE) in children with SLE, as well as the predictive value for TE of persistent versus transient antibodies. In this study of 58 SLE children, LA, aCL, anti-β_2GPI, and antiprothrombin were assessed on at least two occasions (>3 months apart). Outcomes were symptomatic TE (confirmed by objective imaging) identified retrospectively and prospectively. Seven of 58 patients (12%) had 10 TE; 5 patients had TE during prospective follow-up. Persistent LA showed the strongest association with TE ($P <$ 0.0001). Persistent aCL ($P = 0.003$) and anti-β_2GPI ($P = 0.002$) were significantly associated with TE. Persistent or transient LA and anti-β_2GPI showed similar strength of association, while aCL and antiprothrombin were no longer associated with TE. The authors concluded that positivity for multiple aPL subtypes showed stronger associations with TE than for individual aPL subtypes because of improved specificity, that LA is the strongest predictor of the risk of TE, other aPL subtypes provide no additional diagnostic value, and that aCL and antiprothrombin require serial testing, as only persistent antibodies are associated with TE.

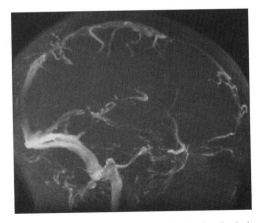

Fig. 1. Angio-MRI showing thrombosis of the superior longitudinal sinus. This 18-year-old boy was affected by APS (secondary to SLE) since age 9.

However, pediatric APS remains relatively rare, as in a large study only in 28 patients out of 1000 with APS, was disease onset before age 15 (with occurrence more frequently in association with SLE or lupus-like disease than in the isolated, primary form) [55].

Other diseases

Juvenile idiopathic arthritis

Several cross-sectional studies have addressed the frequency of aCL in children with juvenile idiopathic arthritis (JIA) giving a global prevalence of around 30% (97 of 320) [11–13,16,45,56]. In the great majority of these studies, no associations between aCL and disease activity have been observed, and no clinical manifestations of APS were detected. There were only two reports of aPL-associated thrombosis in children with JIA [57,58].

aCL, anti-β_2GPI, and LA were prospectively followed in 28 children with JIA. Forty-six percent of patients were positive for aCL already at the first referral, but during follow-up the frequency of aCL positivity decreased to 29%. In contrast, the frequency of positive anti-β_2GPI and LA never exceeded 11%. These observations indicate that aCL are frequently present at the very beginning of JIA, but may not require the presence of β_2GPI for their binding to cardiolipin, similar as postinfectious aPL [59].

Stroke

aPL have been associated with a variety of neurologic manifestations, and central nervous system involvement is frequently present in children with both primary and secondary APS. Several investigators have reported that the prevalence of aPL-associated cerebral ischemia is particularly high in pediatric populations, ranging from 16% to 76% [26,60–65]. Recently, Kenet and colleagues [63] studied the prevalence of thrombophilia risk factors in 58 unrelated children with ischemic stroke compared with 145 controls. All patients were tested for antithrombin III, protein C and protein S deficiencies, the presence of aPL, factor V Leiden, G20210A polymorphism of factor II gene, and C677T polymorphism of 5,10-methylenetetrahydrofolate reductase gene. Fifty-three percent of patients with pediatric stroke were found to have at least one thrombophilia marker compared with only 25.5% of control subjects. The presence of aPL was associated with a greater than sixfold risk of stroke (odds ratio [OR] = 6.08, 95% confidence interval [CI] 1.5–24.3), and the heterozygosity for factor V Leiden increased the risk of stroke by almost fivefold (OR = 4.82, 95% CI 1.4–16.5). These data suggest that the prevalence of thrombophilia markers is increased in children with stroke compared with control subjects; specifically, factor V Leiden and aPL contribute significantly to stroke occurrence.

Thrombosis of the cerebral sinuses has been observed in both primary and secondary APS [66]. A large Canadian study determined the risk factors for sinovenous thrombosis in 160 children [29]. The risk factors were age dependent, often multiple, and different from those reported in adults. Head and neck infections predominated in preschool children, whereas chronic diseases such as connective tissue disorders were more frequent in older children. Risk factors that are common in adults such as pregnancy, cancer, and use of oral contraceptives were rare in this study. Tests for prothrombotic disorders were performed in 123 patients; 32% of them had at least one abnormality. The presence of aCL was the most frequent acquired disorder (10 of 123). In view of these results, the screening of all children with unexplained ischemic stroke or sinovenous thrombosis for aPL might be justified.

Epilepsy

Recent case reports and case series suggest a potential role for aPL in the development of childhood seizure disorder [67–69]. Angelini and colleagues [70] reported persistent aPL positivity in three of 23 children with partial epileptic seizures. In a control group of 40 age- and sex-matched children with other neurologic diseases, no patient was positive for LA, and none was positive for aPL. In another study, the prevalence of aCL and antinuclear (but not glutamic acid decarboxylase) antibodies was higher in a group of epileptic children than in controls [71]. In a prospective study, aPL were tested in 142 pediatric patients with epilepsy [72]. Fifteen (10.6%) were positive for aCL and 25 (17.6%) for anti-β2GPI. The frequency of antiprothrombin antibodies positivity in tested patients was 20% (18 of 90). In total, nearly 30% of patients in this study tested positive for at least one subtype of aPL, and a possible role in the pathogenesis of some forms of epilepsy was hypothesized. Interestingly, antibody positivity tended to correlate with frequency of seizures: in patients who were antibody-positive, there were more subjects with more than one seizure per day. Another study has independently confirmed these findings: in a study of 50 children and 20 healthy subjects, a higher frequency of aPL was found in the study group (44%) compared with controls (10%) [69].

Other neurologic disorders

The prevalence of aPL in neurologic diseases other than stroke has not been extensively studied in childhood, although this issue is of interest in view of possible differences to the adult population. Chorea has been described as an isolated clinical manifestation in children with aPL or in association with SLE [73–79], and there are some data that suggest the association between migraine and aPL in children [75,80]. Although one study [81] showed the presence of LA and aCL in four of nine children with Tourette's syndrome, another larger study showed a non significant increase in prevalence of aPL in 21 children tested in comparaison to healthy controls [19]. Finally, there are yet no data on the presence of more subtle neurologic manifestations, such as mild cognitive impairment, in children with elevated aPL.

Of interest is a large study by Avčin and colleagues [82], who determined the prevalence and clinical associations of aPL with neuropsychiatric manifestations in a cohort of 137 children with SLE. At the time of diagnosis, 23 of 137 children (17%) with SLE presented with neuropsychiatric manifestations, 83 of 128 (65%) had positive aCL and 22 of 84 (26%) had positive LA. Statistically, there was a significant association between positive LA and cerebrovascular disease ($P = 0.015$). There was a trend toward association between LA and chorea ($P = 0.06$). During follow-up (1–118 months with a mean period of 31 months), neuropsychiatric manifestations occurred in 35 of 137 (26%) children with SLE: headache (16%), psychosis (10%), cognitive disfunction (9%), cerebrovascular disease (5%), seizures and mood disorders (3% each), chorea and transverse myelitis (2% each). Persistently positive aCL occurred in 50% (69 of 137) and persistently positive LA in 16% (20 of 125). Among children with SLE and neuropsychiatric manifestations, 49% (17 of 35) had persistently positive aCL and 21% (7 of 34) had persistently positive LA. This study showed a statistically significant association between persistently positive LA and chorea ($P = 0.02$); however, there were only two patients with chorea. These findings suggest an association between positive LA and cerebrovascular disease at the time of SLE diagnosis and between persistently positive LA and chorea over the disease course. No association between aCL or LA and other neuropsychiatric manifestations was demonstrated.

Hematologic diseases, infections, and other disorders

Hematologic abnormalities can occur in APS. Thrombocytopenia can be part of pediatric APS [42,83–85]. Generally it is mild (platelet count between 50–150 × 10^9/L), and there are rarely clinical consequences. In a patient with SLE, it is often difficult to determine whether thrombocytopenia is APS-related, because low platelet counts are a frequent manifestation of the disease itself. Other hematologic abnormalities may occur in children with APS: autoimmune hemolytic anemia, sometimes associated with thrombocytopenia (Evans' syndrome), has also been described in APS secondary to SLE [86]. Interestingly, a paradoxic transient hemorrhagic diathesis has been reported in APS, associated with LA and hypoprothrombinemia, usually preceded by a viral infection [87,88]. This complication has been attributed to the presence of antiprothrombin antibodies that could cause rapid depletion of plasma prothrombin.

Because aPL have been observed in association with various viral infections that are commonly acquired in childhood, a high percentage of aPL positivity might be expected for pediatric population [89]. Indeed, positive aCL were found in 11% of apparently healthy children, which could be partially attributed to some previous infections [10], and Kratz and colleagues

[15] found positive aCL in 30% of 88 children with upper airway infections. The presence of aPL has been reported also in children with acute varicella infection [90], parvovirus B19 infection [91,92] and HIV infection [93]. These findings suggest that aPL positivity should always be verified on at least two occasions, preferably at a time when the child has not had a recent infection, because postinfectious aPL tend to be transient. The majority of infection-associated aPL in children seems to be nonpathogenic, and there are yet no reports of children who suffered from clinical symptoms due to the presence of postinfectious aPL.

The presence of circulating aPL has been observed in a variety of other pediatric autoimmune and nonautoimmune diseases [1] such as insulin-dependent diabetes mellitus [94,95], rheumatic fever [96,97] and Perthes' disease [85]. In most of these conditions, APS is unusual and the significance of aPL should be further confirmed. Skin manifestations of aPL have not been extensively investigated in childhood, but in clinical practice many aPL positive children present with chronically cold hands and livedo reticularis. aPL have been studied also in children with atopic dermatitis [98]. Surprisingly, high frequency of IgG anti-β_2GPI were found with levels comparable to that in adult patients with APS. These anti-β_2GPI may represent exaggerated immune response to nutritional β_2GPI, because the β_2GPI molecule has been remarkably conserved during the evolution of animal species [99]. Ingestion of bovine or some other type of β_2GPI found in different milk or meat products could act as an oral immunization agent and induce transitory production of anti-β_2GPI in infants, in whom the intestinal mucosa is more permissive for large molecules [100]. Ambrozic and colleagues [98] have studied recently aPL in a group of 93 randomly selected children with allergic diseases. A high frequency (42%) of IgG anti-β_2GPI was found in 45 children with atopic dermatitis but none in those with other allergic diseases. These IgG anti-β_2GPI were exclusively of IgG1 subclass and bound to bovine β_2GPI as well, but did not bound to β_2GPI associated with cardiolipin.

Special situations

Neonatal antiphospholipid syndrome

Fetal and neonatal complications such as intrauterine growth restriction and prematurity may occur, despite treatment, in pregnancies of aPL-positive women [101–103].

Evidence exists that in pregnant women with APS, aCL can cross the placenta and be detected in cord blood [104,105]. During 3 months of follow-up of infants born to mothers with APS, it was observed that aCL titers in newborns' sera progressively decreased, and after 6 months the antibodies were undetectable [104]. Transplacental transfer of aPL is not necessarily associated with aPL-related clinical manifestations in newborns. Six studies on the outcome of a total of 269 infants born to mothers with APS have consistently shown that except for prematurity and its potential associated complications (eg, neurologic, pulmonary, ophthalmologic), these neonates had no other clinical manifestations [103,104,106–109]. These are quite surprising results, because it is known that during the first month of life, the risk of thrombotic complications is approximately 40 times greater than at any other age during childhood [110]. Furthermore, premature infants are known to have reduced levels of antithrombin III [111], which may additionally increase the risk of thrombosis. Therefore, one would expect high frequency of neonatal thrombosis in infants born to mothers with APS. The explanation of this discrepancy may be that the aPL IgG subclasses have a different capacity of crossing the placenta, and that the placental transfer of IgG2, which appears to be responsible for most clinical pathogenicity of aPL [112], is actually very low. Alternatively, it can be hypothesized that there are some differences in host susceptibility such as intact vessel wall in the neonates, which do not favor thrombus formation. In general, outcome of infants born to mothers with APS seems to be favorable and similar to their gestational age-matched peers. Isolated case reports of neonatal APS suggest that aPL-related complications can occur also in these infants, but are very rare in comparison to a number of successful aPL pregnancies. It is possible that transplacentally transferred aPL act as a risk factor for neonatal thrombosis, but alone they are apparently unable to induce thrombotic process in uninjured vessels.

There is, however, an increasing number of case reports describing neonates or infants who have suffered from aPL-associated thrombosis. At least seven infants had been reported with aPL-related cerebral ischemia. Silver and colleagues [113] described two infants with middle cerebral artery infarction whose mothers had elevated aCL after delivery. They hypothesized that maternal aCL might have been responsible for intrauterine thromboembolic stroke, but their conclusions were invalidated by the delay between delivery and the laboratory examinations. Teyssier and colleagues [114] reported the occurrence of cerebral ischemia and bilateral massive adrenal hemorrhage in a neonate who was aCL-positive during the neonatal period and 7 months later. De Klerk and colleagues [115] described a LA-positive neonate, who had middle cerebral artery infarct and was born to an apparently healthy mother. Recently, neonatal cerebral ischemia with elevated maternal and infant aCL have been reported in three additional cases [116,117]. Several reports have described neonatal APS cases with other complications including aortic thromboses [118,119], renal vein thrombosis [120], mesenteric thrombosis [121], Blalock-Taussig shunt thrombosis [122], and a neonatal catastrophic APS with multiple thromboses [123]. Additionally, Hage and colleagues [124] described a case of hydrops fetalis with fetal renal vein thrombosis, and suggested that transplacentally transferred maternal aPL may induce typical complications already in the fetus.

In conclusion, the precise risk of thrombosis in infants born to a mother with APS is probably low, but it seems necessary to survey these infants closely. These babies should be monitored for aPL-related clinical manifestations, at least until transplacentally acquired aPL become undetectable [103]. Additionally, aPL should be tested in all newborns with unexplained vascular thrombosis and in their mothers.

An international registry on infants born to mothers with APS has been undertaken as part of the Euro-APL Forum [102]. Its aims are (1) to investigate the presence of aPL in the newborns, and study their relationships with the mothers' clinical, biologic, and therapeutical status; and (2) to evaluate the antibody disappearance and the consequences of the antibody presence on the child's evolution. Any center following women with high-risk pregnancies can participate. This registry is a prospective, multicentric study that aims to follow a cohort of infants born to mothers with APS from birth to the age of 5 years. It will include all consecutive infants born from mothers with APS, fulfilling the recent Sydney consensus criteria [125]. Inclusion can be done at any time during pregnancy until day 3 after birth. Parental consent will be needed. Data are collected at birth, with two forms for the mother and two for the child (clinical and biologic data). General information will include clinical background, APS symptoms, treatment before and during pregnancy, fetal development, pregnancy outcome, pathologic study of the placenta, aPL at diagnosis and subsequently (before pregnancy, during first trimester, and peripartum). The first neonatal examination will be clinical and immuno/hematologic: complete blood count, aPL detected either by cordocentesis or during the first week of life. Clinical and biologic follow-up data will be collected at each examination set up by national pediatric health rules, with a suggested time frame of visits at 1 to 3 months, 9 to 12 months, 24 months, and at 5 to 6 years of age. Additional data will be collected at any medical event possibly related to aPL. Special focus will be on growth and neurodevelopmental milestones. The immunologic aPL follow-up will be realized (even if the detection was initially negative) at 1 to 3 and 6 to 9 months. If aPL persist at 1 year, a clinical and immunologic examination is suggested every 6 months until negative. Any thrombotic episode will be documented by the appropriate exams such as Doppler or MRI.

Up to now, 64 mother/baby pairs have been included in the study. Most of the pregnant women (80%) had primary APS. A high rate of prematurity (12 of 64 babies, 18.7%) was observed; intrauterine growth restriction was observed in 12 of 64 neonates (19%). At birth, aPL were present in 36.5% of babies: LA in 19%, aCL in 12.5%, anti-β2-GPI in 26% and anti-prothrombin antibodies in 8.5% of the babies tested. Comparing the antibodies present in the children at birth and their mothers, unexpected discrepancies in six neonates were found, with presence of aPL not detected in mothers. No postnatal thrombosis, autoimmune disease, or hospitalization were reported. Interestingly, among the 19 babies with clinical evaluation after 1 year of age, two of them had an abnormal behavior, one of them diagnosed as a probable autism. They had no aPL in their sera. The postnatal immunologic follow-up showed that of the 14 aPL-positive babies at birth, 8 became negative at 3 months and 6 were still positive between 3 to 18 months. Surprisingly, in eight initially aPL-negative babies, aPL developed at 3 to 4 months and were still present between 6 to 18 months.

Catastrophic antiphospholipid syndrome

The term "catastrophic" has been used to describe the severity of APS symptomatology; this syndrome has been occasionally reported in children as well [33,126–130]. Asherson and colleagues [128] reviewed 80 patients with catastrophic APS: in four cases, patients were ≤16 years of age. Catastrophic APS is defined as clinical involvement of at least three different organ systems over a period of days or weeks, with histopathologic evidence of multiple occlusions of large or, more often, small vessels [131]. Acute microangiopathy can affect small vessels of multiple organs, including most frequently the kidney, the lung, the central nervous system, the heart, and the skin. Disseminated intravascular coagulation is reported in 25% of cases and mortality rate is 50%. The death is usually caused by multiorgan failure. Some authors have determined precipiting factors for catastrophic APS: infections, surgical procedures, neoplasms, lupus flares, withdrawal of warfarin therapy, and the use of oral contraceptives [132].

Atypical antiphospholipid syndrome in chilhood (acquired coagulation factor inhibitors)

In children, two types of rare APS can induce severe complications. The acquired hypoprothrombinemia–lupus anticoagulant syndrome is a condition that is paradoxically characterized by a bleeding tendency and not by thrombosis, and by the presence of circulating high-affinity antibodies against prothrombin, hypoprothrombinemia, and bleeding. It is often preceded by a viral infection, and has been described in the pediatric age as well as in adults [88,133–135]. Becton and colleagues [88] described sudden onset of bleeding in six previously healthy children due to transient LA and hypoprothrombinemia. Epistaxis was most common, and one child presented with hemarthrosis. Corticosteroid treatment was effective.

Another condition associated with acquired coagulation factor inhibitors, and peculiar to the pediatric age, is that seen after acute varicella virus infection [136]. Postvaricella purpura fulminans or thrombosis have been reported in childhood. Varicella-induced antiprotein S autoantibodies associated with aPL lead to acquired transient decrease in protein S and thromboses [137,138]. Disseminated intravascular coagulation may coexist, resulting in hemorrage [138]. LA and aCL have been identified also in children with this complication, but the specificity of these aPL has not be demonstrated. Additionally, some authors described a significantly increased prevalence of LA and reduced concentration of free protein S in 17 healthy children with acute varicella infection [90]. These findings suggest that varicella virus infection is characterized by a marked hypercoagulability state.

Differential diagnosis

In the differential diagnosis, several conditions have to be ruled out for a child with unexplained thrombosis, including genetic defects, metabolic disorders, myeloproliferative disorders, systemic diseases, and drug-induced thrombosis. A careful history, physical examination, and appropriate laboratory tests are essential to make the correct diagnosis. Diseases and treatments associated with unexplained venous and arterial thrombosis in childhood include Protein C deficiency, Protein S deficiency, antithrombin III deficiency, factor V Leiden mutation (activated protein C resistance), homocysteinemia, myeloproliferative disorders, nephrotic syndrome, systemic vasculitis, Behçet's syndrome, estrogen-containing oral contraceptives, and heparin-induced thrombosis [139].

Treatment

Lack of prospective, randomized, controlled treatment trials has led to considerable debate on the appropriate management of children with aPL, and many clinical questions still remain unanswered. Asymptomatic children, in whom aPL were incidentally found, only rarely develop thrombotic complications. Because of the low thrombosis risk, it is generally assumed that these children do not need any prophylactic treatment [1,2]. The usefulness of aspirin prophylaxis in asymptomatic children with aPL is not known; however, it is usually not recommended because of the increased risk for hemorrhage during play and sports. The optimal management of adolescents with aPL should also include the removal of risk factors such as smoking and oral contraception. Recent data suggest a higher risk of thrombosis in children with elevated aPL and underlying systemic autoimmune disease, such as SLE or lupus-like disease [55]. Low-dose aspirin (at the antiplatelet dosage of 3–5 mg/kg/d) may be considered to be appropriate thromboprophylaxis in these patients, especially when other risk factors are present. The presence of aPL could suggest alternative therapeutic approaches (ie, other antiaggregation, or even anticoagulation) in difficult cases with neurologic involvement or in patients nonresponsive to currently used conventional treatments.

Treatment of the acute thrombotic event in children with APS is no different from that usually given to pediatric patients with venous or arterial thrombosis in the absence of aPL. Patients are anticoagulated with heparin followed by oral anticoagulants. There is general agreement that long-term anticoagulation is needed in children who experienced an aPL-related thrombosis to prevent recurrences, but there is no consensus about the duration and intensity of this therapy. The localization of the thrombosis (ie, venous versus arterial) might be important in deciding on the intensity and duration of treatment. Given that the risk of recurrence might be lower in aPL-positive children compared with adults, and considering the higher risk of hemorrhage during physical activity, it was suggested to perform intermediate-intensity anticoagulation therapy targeted at an international normalized ratio of 2.0 to 2.5 in pediatric patients who have experienced an aPL-related thrombosis [1,2]. In the absence of reliable data, the type and duration of treatment cannot be rationally determined. Therefore, children are normally treated according to the clinical judgment of their physicians, and receive different treatments at different times.

Conclusion: future projects

A register for pediatric patients with APS (Ped-APS Register) has been established in 2004 as a collaborative project of the European Forum on Antiphospholipid Antibodies (Euro-aPL Forum) and the Lupus Working Group of the Pediatric Rheumatology European Society. Its aim is to obtain more generalizable data on the associations of aPL with clinical manifestations in childhood, specificity of aPL in pediatric APS, impact of treatment and long-term outcome of pediatric APS. It is an Internet-based register that allows multicenter data collection, and may be freely consulted at the official Web site of the Euro-aPL Forum (http://www.med.ub.es/MIMMUN/FORUM/PEDIATRIC.HTM). To be eligible for enrollment into this registry, the patient must meet the preliminary criteria for the classification of pediatric APS and the onset of APS must have occurred before the patient's 18th birthday. Exclusion criteria for enrollment into the Ped-APS Register are (1) infants born to mothers with APS and (2) infants with congenital thrombophilia. It is expected that periodic analysis of these data will allow us to increase our knowledge of this condition and to develop a consensus criteria for the classification of pediatric APS.

Summary

APS is rare in the pediatric age, but it represents an interesting phenomenon because most of the known "second hit" risk factors such as atherosclerosis, smoking, hypertension, contraceptive hormonal treatment, and pregnancy are not present in childhood. This could also be the reason for the prevalence of some clinical manifestations rather than others in PAPS. On the other hand, the increased frequency of infectious processes in the childhood age is likely responsible for the relatively high prevalence of non-pathogenic and transient aPL. Such points raise the problem of a different diagnosis or monitoring approach in pediatric APS. Of particular interest is the special entity of neonatal APS, which represents an in vivo model of acquired autoimmune disease, in which transplacentally acquired aPL cause thrombosis in the newborn. International registries for pediatric and neonatal APS are currently in place; epidemiologic, clinical, and laboratory research will help to shed light on all the still obscure aspects of this fascinating but rare disorder in the very young. Finally, treatment is less aggressive overall in pediatric APS, given the reluctance to anticoagulate children over the long term. Studies on the outcome of pediatric APS and the relative risks of prolonged anticoagulation in children are necessary to determine the type and duration of anticoagulation therapy.

References

[1] Ravelli A, Martini A. Antiphospholipid antibody syndrome in pediatric patients. Rheum Dis Clin North Am 1997;23(3):657–76.

[2] Tucker LB. Antiphospholipid antibodies and antiphospholipid syndromes in children. In: Khamashta MA, editor. Hughes syndrome, antiphospholipid syndrome. London: Springer; 2000. p. 155–66.

[3] Tucker LB. Antiphospholipid syndrome in childhood: the great unknown. Lupus 1994; 3(5):367–9.

[4] Szer IS. Clinical development in the management of lupus in the neonate, child, and adolescent. Curr Opin Rheumatol 1998;10(5):431–4.

[5] Lee T, von Scheven E, Sandborg C. Systemic lupus erythematosus and antiphospholipid syndrome in children and adolescents. Curr Opin Rheumatol 2001;13(5):415–21.

[6] Ravelli A, Martini A. Antiphospholipid syndrome. Pediatr Clin North Am 2005;52(2): 469–91.

[7] Avčin T, Cimaz R, Meroni PL. Recent advances in antiphospholipid antibodies and antiphospholipid syndromes in pediatric poplulations. Lupus 2002;11(1):4–11.

[8] Male C, Lechner K, Eichinger S, et al. Clinical significance of lupus anticoagulants in children. J Pediatr 1999;134(2):199–205.

[9] Rapizzi E, Ruffatti A, Tonello M, et al. Correction for age of anticardiolipin antibodies cut-off points. J Clin Lab Anal 2000;14(3):87–90.

[10] Avčin T, Ambrozic A, Kuhar M, et al. Anticardiolipin and anti-β2 glycoprotein I antibodies in sera of 61 apparently healthy children at regular preventive visits. Rheumatol 2001;40(5):565–73.

[11] Caporali R, Ravelli A, De Gennaro F, et al. Prevalence of anticardiolipin antibodies in juvenile arthritis. Ann Rheum Dis 1991;50(9):599–601.

[12] Siamopoulou-Mavridou A, Mavridis AK, Terzoglou C, et al. Autoantibodies in Greek juvenile chronic arthritis patients. Clin Exp Rheumatol 1991;9(6):647–52.

[13] Gattorno M, Buoncompagni A, Molinari AC, et al. Antiphospholipid antibodies in paediatric systemic lupus erythematosus, juvenile chronic arthritis and overlap syndromes: SLE patients with both lupus anticoagulant and high-titre anticardiolipin antibodies are at risk for clinical manifestations related to the antiphospholipid syndrome. Br J Rheumatol 1995; 34(9):873–81.

[14] Kontiainen S, Miettinen A, Seppälä I, et al. Antiphospholipid antibodies in children. Acta Paediatr 1996;85(5):614–5.

[15] Kratz C, Mauz-Körholz C, Kruck H, et al. Detection of antiphospholipid antibodies in children and adolescents. Pediatr Hematol Oncol 1998;15(4):325–32.

[16] Serra CRB, Rodrigues SH, Silva NP, et al. Clinical significance of anticardiolipin antibodies in juvenile idiopathic arthritis. Clin Exp Rheumatol 1999;17(3):375–80.

[17] Gallistl S, Muntean W, Leschnik B, et al. PTT values in healthy children than in adults: no single cause. Thromb Res 1997;88(4):355–9.

[18] Siemens HJG, Gutsche S, Brückner S, et al. Antiphospholipid antibodies in children without and in adults with and without thrombophilia. Thromb Res 2000;98(4):241–7.

[19] Casais P, Meschengieser SS, Gennari LC, et al. Morbidity of lupus anticoagulants in children: a single institution experience. Thromb Res 2004;114(4):245–9.

[20] Singer HS, Krumholz A, Giuliano J, et al. Antiphospholipid antibodies: an epiphenomenon in Tourette syndrome. Mov Disord 1997;12(5):738–42.

[21] Manco-Johnson MJ, Nuss R. Lupus anticoagulant in children with thrombosis. Am J Hematol 1995;48(4):240–3.

[22] Von Scheven E, Athreya B, Rose CD, et al. Clinical characteristics of antiphospholipid antibody syndrome in children. J Pediatr 1996;129(3):339–45.

[23] Nuss R, Hays T, Chudgar U, et al. Antiphospholipid antibodies and coagulation regulatory protein abnormalities in children with pulmonary emboli. J Pediatr Hematol Oncol 1997; 19(3):202–7.

[24] Brady L, Magilavy D, Black DD. Portal vein thrombosis associated with antiphospholipid antibodies in a child. J Pediatr Gastroenterol Nutr 1996;23(4):470–3.

[25] Falcini F, Taccetti G, Trapani S, et al. Primary antiphospholipid syndrome: a report of two pediatric cases. J Rheumatol 1991;18(7):1085–7.

[26] Angelini L, Ravelli A, Caporali R, et al. High prevalence of antiphospholipid antibodies in children with idiopathic cerebral ischemia. Pediatrics 1994;94(4):500–3.

[27] Di Nucci GD, Mariani G, Arcieri P, et al. Antiphospholipid syndrome in young patients. Two cases of cerebral ischemic accidents. Eur J Pediatr 1995;154(4):334.

[28] Olson JC, Konkol RJ, Gill JC, et al. Childhood stroke and lupus anticoagulant. Pediatr Neurol 1994;10(1):54–7.

[29] DeVeber G, Andrew M, Adams C, et al. Cerebral sinovenous thrombosis in children. N Engl J Med 2001;345(6):417–23.

[30] Heller C, Heinecke A, Junker R, et al. Cerebral venous thrombosis in children: a multifactorial origin. Circulation 2003;108(11):1362–7.

[31] Hasegawa M, Yamashita J, Yamashima T, et al. Spinal cord infarction associated with primary antiphospholipid syndrome in a young child. J Neurosurg 1993;79(3): 446–50.

[32] Ohtomo Y, Matsubara T, Nishizawa K, et al. Nephropathy and hypertension as manifestations in a 13-y-old girl with primary antiphospholipid syndrome. Acta Paediatr 1998; 87(8):903–7.

[33] Falcini F, Taccetti G, Ermini M, et al. Catastrophic antiphospholipid antibody syndrome in pediatric systemic lupus erythematosus. J Rheumatol 1997;24(2):389–92.

[34] Avčin T, Cimaz R, Meroni PL. Do we need international consensus statement on classification criteria for the antiphospholipid syndrome in paediatric population? Lupus 2001; 10(12):897–8.

[35] Gattorno M, Falcini F, Ravelli A, et al. Outcome of primary antiphospholipid syndrome in childhood. Lupus 2003;12(6):449–53.

[36] Tan EM, Cohen AS, Fries JF, et al. The 1982 revised criteria for the classification of systemic lupus erythematosus. Arthritis Rheum 1982;25(11):1271–7.

[37] Gomez JA, Martin H, Amigo MC, et al. Long-term follow-up in 90 patients with primary antiphospolilid syndrom (PAPS). Do they develop lupus? Arthritis Rheum 2001; 44(Suppl):S146.

[38] Shergy WJ, Kredich DW, Pisetsky DS. The relationship of anticardiolipin antibodies to disease manifestations in pediatric systemic lupus erythematosus. J Rheumatol 1988;15(9): 1389–94.

[39] Montes de Oca MA, Babron MC, Bletry O, et al. Thrombosis in systemic lupus erythematosus: a French collaborative study. Arch Dis Child 1991;66(6):713–7.

[40] Molta C, Meyer O, Dosquet C, et al. Childhood-onset systemic lupus erythematosus: anti-phospholipid antibodies in 37 patients and their first degree relatives. Pediatrics 1993;92(6): 849–53.

[41] Ravelli A, Caporali R, Di Fuccia G, et al. Anticardiolipin antibodies in pediatric systemic lupus erythematosus. Arch Pediatr Adolesc Med 1994;148(4):398–402.

[42] Seaman DE, Londino V, Kent Kwoh C, et al. Antiphospholipid antibodies in pediatric systemic lupus erythematosus. Pediatrics 1995;96(6):1040–5.

[43] Massengill SF, Hedrick C, Ayoub EM, et al. Antiphospholipid antibodies in pediatric lupus nephritis. Am J Kidney Dis 1997;29(3):355–61.

[44] Berube C, Mitchell L, Silverman E, et al. The relationship of antiphospholipid antibodies to thromboembolic events in pediatric patients with systemic lupus erythematosus. Pediatr Res 1998;44(3):351–6.

[45] Gedalia A, Molin A, Garcia CO, et al. Anticardiolipin antibodies in childhood rheumatic disorders. Lupus 1998;7(8):551–3.

[46] von Scheven E, Glidden DV, Elder ME. Anti-beta2-glycoprotein I antibodies in pediatric systemic lupus erythematosus and antiphospholipid syndrome. Arthritis Rheum 2002; 47(4):414–20.

[47] Campos LM, Kiss MH, D'Amico EA, et al. Antiphospholipid antibodies and antiphospho lipid syndrome in 57 children and adolescents with systemic lupus erythematosus. Lupus 2003;12(11):820–6.

[48] Levy DM, Massicotte MP, Harvey E, et al. Thromboembolism in paediatric lupus patients. Lupus 2003;12(10):741–6.

[49] Schmugge M, Revel-Vilk S, Hiraki L, et al. Thrombocytopenia and thromboembolism in pediatric systemic lupus erythematosus. J Pediatr 2003;143(5):666–9.

[50] Dungan DD, Jay MS. Stroke in an early adolescent with systemic lupus erythematosus and coexistent antiphospholipid antibodies. Pediatrics 1992;90(1):96–8.

[51] Kwong T, Leonidas JC, Ilowite NT. Asymptomatic superior vena cava thrombosis and pulmonary embolism in an adolescent with SLE and antiphospholipid antibodies. Clin Exp Rheumatol 1994;12(2):215–7.

[52] Baca V, Sanchez-Vaca G, Martinez-Muniz I, et al. Successful treatment of transverse myelitis in a child with systemic lupus erythematosus. Neuropediatrics 1996;27(1):42–4.

[53] Tomizawa K, Sato-Matsumura KC, Kajii N. The coexistence of cutaneous vasculitis and thrombosis in childhood-onset systemic lupus erythematosus with antiphospholipid antibodies. Br J Dermatol 2003;149(2):439–41.

[54] Male C, Foulon D, Hoogendoorn H, et al. Predictive value of persistent versus transient antiphospholipid antibody subtypes for the risk of thrombotic events in pediatric patients with systemic lupus erythematosus. Blood 2005;106(13):4152–8.

[55] Cervera R, Piette JC, Font J, et al. Antiphospholipid syndrome: clinical and immunologic manifestations and patterns of disease expression in a cohort of 1000 patients. Arthritis Rheum 2002;46(4):19–27.

[56] Leak AM, Colaco CB, Isenberg DA. Anticardiolipin and anti-ss DNA antibodies in antinuclear positive juvenile chronic arthritis and other childhood onset rheumatic diseases. Clin Exp Rheumatol 1987;5:18.

[57] Caporali R, Ravelli A, Ramenghi B, et al. Antiphospholipid antibody associated thrombosis in juvenile chronic arthritis. Arch Dis Child 1992;67(11):1384–5.

[58] Andrews A, Hickling P. Thrombosis associated with antiphospholipid antibody in juvenile chronic arthritis. Lupus 1997;6(6):556–7.

[59] Avčin T, Ambrozic A, Bozic B, et al. Estimation of anticardiolipin antibodies, anti-β2 glycoprotein I antibodies and lupus anticoagulant in a prospective longitudinal study of children with juvenile idiopathic arthritis. Clin Exp Rheumatol 2002;20(1):101–8.

[60] Schöning M, Klein R, Krägeloh-Mann I, et al. Antiphospholipid antibodies in cerebrovascular ischemia and stroke in childhood. Neuropediatrics 1994;25(1):8–14.

[61] Takanashi J, Sugita K, Miyazato S, et al. Antiphospholipid antibody syndrome in child-hood strokes. Pediatr Neurol 1995;13(4):323–6.

[62] Baca V, Garcia-Ramirez R, Ramirez-Lacayo M, et al. Cerebral infarction and antiphos-pholipid syndrome in children. J Rheumatol 1996;23(8):1428–31.

[63] Kenet G, Sadetzki S, Murad H, et al. Factor V Leiden and antiphospholipid antibodies are significant risk factors for ischemic stroke in children. Stroke 2000;31(6):1283–8.

[64] Katsarou E, Attilakos A, Fessatou S, et al. Anti-β2 glycoprotein I antibodies and ischemic stroke in a 20-month-old boy. Pediatrics 2003;112(1):188–90.

[65] Ebeling F, Petaja J, Alanko S, et al. Infant stroke and β2 glycoprotein 1 antibodies: six cases. Eur J Pediatr 2003;162(10):678–81.

[66] Uziel Y, Laxer RM, Blaser S, et al. Cerebral vein thrombosis in childhood systemic lupus erythematosus. J Pediatr 1995;126(5):722–7.

[67] Spreafico R, Binelli S, Bruzzone MG, et al. Primary antiphospholipid syndrome (PAPS) and isolated partial seizures in adolescence. A case report. Ital J Neurol Sci 1994;15(6): 297–301.

[68] Yoshimura K, Konishi T, Kotani H, et al. Prevalence of positive anticardiolipin antibody in benign infantile convulsion. Brain Dev 2001;23(5):317–20.

[69] Eriksson K, Peltola J, Keranen T, et al. High prevalence of antiphospholipid antibodies in children with epilepsy: a controlled study of 50 cases. Epilepsy Res 2001;46(2):129–37.

[70] Angelini L, Granata T, Zibordi F, et al. Partial seizures associated with antiphospholipid antibodies in childhood. Neuropediatrics 1998;29(5):249–53.

[71] Verrotti A, Greco R, Altobelli E, et al. Anticardiolipin, glutamic acid decarboxylase, and antinuclear antibodies in epileptic patients. Clin Exp Med 2003;3(1):32–6.

[72] Cimaz R, Romeo A, Scarano A, et al. Prevalence of anti-cardiolipin, anti-β2 Glyco-protein I, and anti-prothrombin antibodies in young patients with epilepsy. Epilepsia 2002;43(1):52–9.

[73] Vlachoyiannopoulos PG, Dimou G, Siamopoulou-Mavridou A. Chorea as a manifestation of the antiphospholipid syndrome in childhood. Clin Exp Rheumatol 1991;9(3):303–5.

[74] Besbas N, Damarguc I, Ozen S, et al. Association of antiphospholipid antibodies with sys-temic lupus erythematosus in a child presenting with chorea: a case report. Eur J Pediatr 1994;153(12):891–3.

[75] Angelini L, Zibordi F, Zorzi G, et al. Neurological disorders, other than stroke, associated with antiphospholipid antibodies in childhood. Neuropediatrics 1996;27(3):149–53.

[76] Okun MS, Jummani RR, Carney PR. Antiphospholipid-associated recurrent chorea and ballism in a child with cerebral palsy. Pediatr Neurol 2000;23(1):62–3.

[77] Al-Matar M, Jaimes J, Malleson P. Chorea as the presenting clinical feature of primary antiphospholipid syndrome in childhood. Neuropediatrics 2000;31(2):107–8.

[78] Okun MS, Jummani RR, Carney PR. Antiphospholipid-associated recurrent chorea and ballism in a child with cerebral palsy. Pediatr Neurol 2000;23(1):62–3.

[79] Besbas N, Anlar B, Apak A, et al. Optic neuropathy in primary antiphospholipid syndrome in childhood. J Child Neurol 2001;16(9):690–3.

[80] Avčin T, Markelj G, Niksic V, et al. Estimation of antiphospholipid antibodies in a prospec-tive longitudinal study of children with migraine. Cephalalgia 2004;24(10):831–7.

[81] Toren P, Toren A, Weizman A, et al. Tourette's Disorder: is there an association with the antiphospholipid syndrome? Biol Psychiatry 1994;35(7):495–8.

[82] Avcin T, Benseler SM, Tyrrell PN, et al. Longitudinal follow-up study of antiphospholipid antibodies and associated neuropsychiatric manifestations in 137 children with systemic lu-pus erythematosus [abstract F29]. In: Program book supplement of the American College of Rheumatology/Association of Reumatology Health Professionals Annual Scientific Meeting, San Diego, CA. 2005. p. 30–1.

[83] Sakai M, Shirahata A, Akatsuka J, et al. Antiphospholipid antibodies in children with idiopathic thrombocytopenic purpura. Rinsho Ketsueki 2002;43(9):821–7.

[84] Toren A, Toren P, Many A, et al. Spectrum of clinical manifestations of antiphospholipid antibodies in childhood and adolescence. Pediatr Hematol Oncol 1993;10(4):311–5.

[85] Ura Y, Hara T, Mori Y, et al. Development of Perthes' disease in a 3-year-old boy with idiopathic thrombocytopenic purpura and antiphospholipid antibodies. Pediatr Hematol Oncol 1992;9(1):77–80.

[86] Avčin T, Jazbec J, Kuhar M, et al. Evans syndrome associated with antiphospholipid antibodies. J Pediatr Hematol Oncol 2003;25(9):73–4.

[87] Lee MT, Nardi MA, Hadzi-Nesic J, et al. Transient hemorrhagic diathesis associated with an inhibitor of prothrombin with lupus anticoagulant in a 1-year-old girl: report of a case and review of the literature. Am J Hematol 1996;51(4):307–14.

[88] Becton DL, Stine KC. Transient lupus anticoagulants associated with hemorrhage rather than thrombosis: the hemorrhagic lupus anticoagulant syndrome. J Pediatr 1997; 130(6):998–1000.

[89] Vaarala O, Palosuo T, Kleemola M, et al. Anticardiolipin response in acute infections. Clin Immunol Immunopathol 1986;41(1):8–15.

[90] Kurugol Z, Vardar F, Ozkinay F, et al. Lupus anticoagulant and protein S deficiency in otherwise healthy children with acute varicella infection. Acta Pediatr 2000;89(5):1186–9.

[91] Lehmann HW, Plentz A, Von Landenberg P, et al. Intravenous immunoglobulin treatment of four patients with juvenile polyarticular arthritis associated with persistent parvovirus B19 infection and antiphospholipid antibodies. Arthritis Res Ther 2004;6(1):R1–6.

[92] Von Landenberg P, Lehmann HW, Knoll A, et al. Antiphospholipid antibodies in pediatric and adult patients with rheumatic disease are associated with parvovirus B19 infection. Arthritis Rheum 2003;48(7):1939–47.

[93] Carreno L, Monteagudo I, Lopez-Longo FJ, et al. Anticardiolipin antibodies in pediatric patients with human immunodeficiency virus. J Rheumatol 1994;21(7):1344–6.

[94] Lorini R, d'Annunzio G, Montecucco C, et al. Anticardiolipin antibodies in children and adolescents with insulin-dependent diabetes mellitus. Eur J Pediatr 1995;154(2):105–8.

[95] Best IM, Anyadike NC, Bumpers HL. The antiphospholipid syndrome in a teenager with miscarriages, thrombosis, and diabetes mellitus. Am Surgeon 2000;66(8):748–50.

[96] Figueroa F, Berrios X, Gutierrez M, et al. Anticardiolipin antibodies in acute rheumatic fever. J Rheumatol 1992;19(8):1175–80.

[97] Narin N, Kutukculer N, Narin F, et al. Anticardiolipin antibodies in acute rheumatic fever and chronic rheumatic heart disease: is there a significant association? Clin Exp Rheumatol 1996;14(5):567–9.

[98] Ambrozic A, Avčin T, Ichikawa K, et al. Anti-β2-glycoprotein I antibodies in children with atopic dermatitis. Int Immunol 2002;14(7):823–30.

[99] Matsuura E, Igarashi M, Igarashi Y, et al. Molecular definition of human b2-glycoprotein I (b2-GPI) by cDNA cloning and interspecies differences of b2-GPI in alteration of anticardiolipin binding. Int Immunol 1991;3(12):1217–21.

[100] Avčin T, Kveder T, Rozman B. The antiphospholipid syndrome [letter]. N Engl J Med 2002;347(2):145–6.

[101] Backos M, Rai R, Baxter N, et al. Pregnancy complications in women with recurrent miscarriage associated with antiphospholipid antibodies treated with low dose aspirin and heparin. Br J Obstet Gynaecol 1999;106(2):102–7.

[102] Boffa MC, Aurousseau MH, Lachassinne E, et al. European register of babies born to mothers with antiphospholipid syndrome. Lupus 2004;13(9):713–7.

[103] Motta M, Tincani A, Lojacono A, et al. Neonatal outcome in patients with rheumatic disease. Lupus 2004;13(9):718–23.

[104] Zurgil N, Bakimer R, Tincani A, et al. Detection of anti-phospholipid and anti-DNA antibodies and their idiotypes in newborns of mothers with anti-phospholipid syndrome and SLE. Lupus 1993;2(4):233–7.

[105] Cohen SB, Goldenberg M, Rabinovici J, et al. Anti-cardiolipin antibodies in fetal blood and amniotic fluid derived from patients with the anti-phospholipid syndrome. Hum Reprod 2000;15(5):1170–2.

[106] Pollard JK, Scott JR, Branch DW. Outcome of children born to women treated during pregnancy for the antiphospholipid syndrome. Obstet Gynecol 1992;80(3):365–8.

[107] Botet F, Romera G, Montagut P, et al. Neonatal outcome in women treated for the antiphospholipid syndrome during pregnancy. J Perinat Med 1997;25(2):192–6.

[108] Ruffatti A, Dalla Barba B, Del Ross T, et al. Outcome of fifty-five newborns of antiphospholipid antibody-positive mothers treated with calcium heparin during pregnancy. Clin Exp Rheumatol 1998;16(5):605–10.

[109] Brewster JA, Shaw NJ, Farquharson RG. Neonatal and pediatric outcome of infants born to mothers with antiphospholipid syndrome. J Perinat Med 1999;27(3):183–7.

[110] Andrew M, David M, Adams M, et al. Venous thromboembolic complications (VTE) in children: first analyses of the Canadian Registry of VTE. Blood 1994;83(5):1251–7.

[111] Andrew M, Paes B, Milner R, et al. Development of the human coagulation system in the healthy premature infant. Blood 1988;72(5):1651–7.

[112] Sammaritano LR, Ng S, Sobel R, et al. Anticardiolipin IgG subclasses: association of IgG2 with arterial and/or venous thrombosis. Arthritis Rheum 1997;40(11):1998–2006.

[113] Silver RK, MacGregor SN, Pasternak JF, et al. Fetal stroke associated with elevated maternal anticardiolipin antibodies. Obstet Gynecol 1992;80(3):497–9.

[114] Teyssier G, Gautheron V, Absi L, et al. Anticorps anticardiolipine, ischemie cerebrale et hemorragie surrenalienne chez un nouveau-né. Arch Pediatr 1995;2(11):1086–8.

[115] de Klerk OL, de Vries TW, Sinnige LGF. An unusual cause of neonatal seizures in a newborn infant. Pediatrics 1997;100(4):E8.

[116] Akanli LF, Trasi SS, Thuraisamy K, et al. Neonatal middle cerebral artery infarction: association with elevated maternal anticardiolipin antibodies. Am J Perinatol 1998;15(6): 399–402.

[117] Chow G, Mellor D. Neonatal cerebral ischaemia with elevated maternal and infant anticardiolipin antibodies. Dev Med Child Neurol 2000;42(6):412–3.

[118] Finazzi G, Cortelazzo S, Viero P, et al. Maternal lupus anticoagulant and fatal neonatal thrombosis. Thromb Haemost 1987;57(2):238.

[119] Sheridan-Pereira M, Porreco RP, Hays T, et al. Neonatal aortic thrombosis associated with the lupus anticoagulant. Obstet Gynecol 1988;71(6):1016–8.

[120] Contractor S, Hiatt M, Kosmin M, et al. Neonatal thrombosis with anticardiolipin antibody in baby and mother. Am J Perinatol 1992;9(5–6):409–10.

[121] Navarro F, Dona-Naranjo MA, Villanueva I. Neonatal antiphospholipid syndrome. J Rheumatol 1997;24(6):1240–1.

[122] Deally C, Hancock BJ, Giddins N, et al. Primary antiphospholipid syndrome: a cause of catastrophic shunt thrombosis in the newborn. J Cardiovasc Surg (Torino) 1999; 40(2):261–4.

[123] Tabbutt S, Griswold WR, Ogino MT, et al. Multiple thromboses in a premature infant associated with maternal phospholipid antibody syndrome. J Perinatol 1994;14(1):66–70.

[124] Hage ML, Liu R, Marcheschi DG, et al. Fetal renal vein thrombosis, hydrops fetalis, and maternal lupus anticoagulant. A case report. Prenat Diagn 1994;14(9):873–7.

[125] Miyakis S, Lockshin MD, Atsumi T, et al. International consensus statement on an update of the classification criteria for definite antiphospholipid syndrome (APS). J Thromb Haemost 2006;4(2):295–306.

[126] Orsino A, Schneider R, DeVeber G, et al. Childhood acute myelomonocytic leukemia (AML-M4) presenting as catastrophic antiphospholipid syndrome. J Pediatr Hematol Oncol 2004;26(5):327–30.

[127] Schaar CG, Ronday KH, Boets EPM, et al. Catastrophic manifestation of the antiphospholipid syndrome. J Rheumatol 1999;26(10):2261–4.

[128] Asherson RA, Cervera R, Piette JC, et al. Catastrophic antiphospholipid syndrome: clues to the pathogenisis from a serie of 80 patients. Medicine (Baltimore) 2001;80(6):355–77.

[129] Rojas-Rodriguez J, Garcia-Carrasco M, Ramos Casals M, et al. Catastrophic antiphospholipid syndrome: clinical description and triggering factors in eight patients. J Rheumatol 2000;27(1):238–40.

[130] Miyamae T, Imagawa T, Ito S, et al. Effective combination therapy of plasma exchange and subsequent cyclophosphamide pulses for catastrophic antiphospholipid syndrome: a case report. Ryumachi 1999;39(3):391–7.

[131] Asherson RA, Cervera R, Piette JC, et al. Catastrophic antiphospholipid syndrome. Clinical and laboratory features in 50 patients. Medicine (Baltimore) 1998;77(3): 195–207.

[132] Erkan D, Cervera R, Asherson RA. Catastrophic antiphospholipid syndrome. Where do we stand? Arthritis Rheum 2003;48(12):3320–7.

[133] Bernini JC, Buchanan GR, Ashcraft J. Hypoprothrombinemia and severe hemorrhage associated with a lupus anticoagulant. J Pediatr 1993;123(6):937–9.

[134] Eberhard A, Sparling C, Sudbury S, et al. Hypoprothrombinemia in childhood systemic lupus erythematosus. Semin Arthritis Rheum 1994;24(1):12–8.

[135] Hudson N, Duffy CM, Rauch J, et al. Catastrophic hemorrhage in a case of pediatric primary antiphospholipid syndrome and factor II deficiency. Lupus 1997;6(1):68–71.

[136] Josephson C, Nuss R, Jacobson L, et al. The varicella-autoantibody syndrome. Pediatr Res 2001;50(3):345–52.

[137] D'Angelo A, Della Valle P, Crippa L, et al. Brief report: auto-immune protein S deficiency in a boy with severe thromboembolic disease. N Engl J Med 1993;328(24):1753–7.

[138] Kurugol Z, Vardar F, Ozkinay F, et al. Lupus anticoagulant and protein S defiency in a child with postvaricella purpura fulminans or thrombosis. Turk J Pediatr 2001;43(2): 139–42.

[139] Sammaritano LR, Piette JC. Pediatric and familial antiphospholipd syndromes. In: Asherson RA, Cervera R, Piette JC, Shoenfeld Y, editors. The antiphospholipid syndrome II: autoimmune thrombosis. Amsterdam: Elsevier; 2002. p. 297–316.

ELSEVIER
SAUNDERS

Rheum Dis Clin N Am
32 (2006) 575–590

RHEUMATIC
DISEASE CLINICS
OF NORTH AMERICA

Catastrophic Antiphospholipid Syndrome

Ricard Cervera, MD, PhD, FRCP[a],*,
Ronald A. Asherson, MD, FRCP, FACP[b],
Josep Font, MD, PhD, FRCP[a]

[a]Department of Autoimmune Diseases, Hospital Clínic, Villarroel 170,
08036-Barcelona, Catalonia, Spain
[b]Division of Immunology, School of Pathology, University of the Witwatersrand,
Johannesburg, South Africa

The descriptive adjective "catastrophic" was added to the term antiphospholipid syndrome (APS) in 1992 by Asherson [1,2] to highlight an accelerated form of this syndrome resulting in multiorgan failure. Patients with catastrophic APS have in common: clinical evidence of multiple organ involvement developing over a very short period of time; histopathologic evidence of multiple small vessel occlusions; and laboratory confirmation of the presence of antiphospholipid antibodies (aPL), usually in high titer. Furthermore, approximately 60% of the catastrophic episodes are preceded by a precipitating event, mainly infections [1–6].

Although less than 1% of patients with the APS develop this complication [7], its potentially lethal outcome emphasizes its importance in clinical medicine today. The majority of patients with catastrophic APS end up in intensive care units (ICU) with multiorgan failure and, unless the condition is considered in the differential diagnosis by the attending physicians, it may be completely missed, resulting in a disastrous outcome for these patients.

The rarity of this syndrome makes it extraordinarily difficult to study in any systematic way. To correlate all the published case reports as well as newly diagnosed cases from all over the world, an international registry of patients with catastrophic APS ("CAPS Registry") was created in 2000 by the *European Forum on Antiphospholipid Antibodies*, a study group devoted to the development of multicenter projects with large populations of APS patients [8]. Currently, it documents the entire clinical, laboratory, and

* Corresponding author.
E-mail address: rcervera@clinic.ub.es (R. Cervera).

0889-857X/06/$ - see front matter © 2006 Elsevier Inc. All rights reserved.
doi:10.1016/j.rdc.2006.05.002
rheumatic.theclinics.com

therapeutic data of more than 300 patients whose data has been fully registered. This registry can be freely consulted through the Internet at www. med.ub.es/MIMMUN/FORUM/CAPS.HTM.

Furthermore, the heterogeneity of the different clinical forms of presentation led to the development of consensus criteria for the definition and classification of these patients. In September of 2002, a presymposium workshop held during the "Tenth International Congress on aPL" in Taormina, Sicily, Italy, established preliminary criteria for the classification of the catastrophic APS, and were recently published [9] and validated [10].

Pathogenesis

It is still unclear why some patients will develop recurrent thromboses, mainly affecting large vessels, while others develop rapidly recurrent vascular occlusions, predominantly affecting small vessels. Indeed, some of the preceding precipitating or "trigger" factors may be identical in both simple and classic APS patients and in those with catastrophic APS. Clearly, other factors, as yet unidentified, must play important roles.

General factors implicated in the causation of thromboses, including prolonged bed rest, sedentary situations (eg, long-haul flying), dyslipidemias, diabetes mellitus, nephrotic syndrome and obesity, do not seem to be important in its pathogenesis and, interestingly enough, patients suffering from the hereditary coagulopathies (eg, protein C and S or antithrombin III deficiencies and factor V Leiden or prothrombin gene mutations) also do not appear to be prone to this complication. It seems to be a primary "autoimmune" situation associated with high levels of aPL and, in most cases, also accompanied by other severe autoimmune disturbances, such as severe thrombocytopenia or microangiopathic hemolytic anemia, which can complicate the clinical picture, and hence, the diagnosis and treatment.

The occurrence of a systemic inflammatory response syndrome (SIRS), the main clinical manifestation of which is acute respiratory distress syndrome (ARDS), probably results from the liberation of extensive amounts of cytokines and tissue necrosis (usually involving bowel) seen in this condition. It is not seen in other conditions with extensive small vessel involvement (eg, thrombotic thrombocytopenic purpura [TTP]), as they are not accompanied by this extensive necrosis and gangrene seen in the catastrophic APS.

From the CAPS Registry, it can be seen that at least 60% of patients appear to have developed catastrophic APS following an identifiable "trigger" factor, with infections dominating the list (Table 1).

Infections

These include nonspecific viral infections, pneumonias, infected leg ulcers, upper respiratory, urinary, gastrointestinal and cutaneous infections, as well as specific infections such as typhoid fever, malaria, and Dengue

Table 1
Precipitating factors according to the analysis of 250 patients from the "CAPS Registry"

• Unknown	40%
• Infections	22%
• Trauma	14%
• Anticoagulation problems	7.2%
• Neoplasia	6.8%
• Obstetric	4.6%
• Lupus "flares"	3%
• Other[a]	5.5%

[a] These include oral contraceptives, immunization, ovulation induction, and drugs such as danazol and thiazides.

fever, among others. Postulated mechanisms by which infections may cause thrombosis have been a subject of much interest over the past 2 years. An editorial devoted to discuss the potential role of *molecular mimicry* in the pathogenesis of catastrophic APS was published in 2000 [11], and studies undertaken in Shoenfeld's laboratories in Israel by Miri Blank and colleagues have made a significant contribution to the understanding of the many and diverse mechanisms that could be invoked, such as linking the structure and function of β-2 glycoprotein I (β-2GP1) itself (the main antigen against which the aPL are directed), to the role of infection and thrombosis. Credit must also be given to the work of the late Azzudin Gharavi and colleagues [12,13], who identified seven proteins with sequence homology to the GDKU and GDKU2 proteins (which are the major phospholipid binding sites on β-2GP1, and which form part of many human viruses to which humans are exposed). Moreover, immunization of groups of mice with these peptides together with Freund's adjuvant produced high levels of aPL and anti-β-2GP1 antibodies. The finding that ciprofloxacin, a common member of the quinolone family with antibiotic properties that increase production of interleukin (IL)-3, a cytokine deficient in mice with experimental APS as well as in humans with the APS, may benefit mice with experimental APS, is further confirmatory evidence of an infectious etiology in some catastrophic APS patients. These studies on the possible infectious origin of the APS and its catastrophic variant were rewarded with the EULAR Prize in 2005 [14].

Trauma/surgical procedures

Both major (hysterectomy, cholecystectomy, pelvic surgery, cesarean section, and so on) and minor (lung/renal biopsies, dental extraction, dilatation and curettage, needle stick injury, cataract removal) surgical procedures have been reported as "triggers" of catastrophic APS. The mechanisms by which trauma/surgical procedures may initiate catastrophic APS are unknown, but might involve excessive cytokine production affecting endothelial cell function and the expression and upregulation of procoagulant molecules as well as production of tissue factor.

Malignancies

In several patients, malignancies appeared to be associated with the development of catastrophic APS. They included carcinoma of the lung, stomach, colon, and uterus, cholangiocarcinoma of the gall bladder and B-cell lymphoma, among others [15].

Lupus "flares"

The low prevalence of catastrophic APS associated with "lupus" flares is surprising, but makes a case for alternative mechanisms involved in the pathogenesis of this condition other than just the overproduction of antibodies. A possible case can be made for the use of anticoagulant therapy in patients with lupus "flares" who have high levels of aPL and who have not yet experienced any thrombotic episodes.

Warfarin withdrawal/low international normalized ratio

Warfarin withdrawal, before major surgical procedures or minor procedures (eg, biopsies), or because of hemorrhagic complications usually attributable to anticoagulation therapy, may be followed within a short time either by recurrent thrombosis or by catastrophic APS, particularly if other "trigger" factors are also present (eg, underlying carcinoma, infection). This is the so-called *double or treble hit hypothesis*, which applies to any patient with multiorgan failure. Great care should be taken to ensure that these patients are covered during these procedures by adequate parenteral anticoagulation.

Kitchens hypothesis

Kitchens [16] advanced the hypothesis that large clots themselves may be responsible for the ongoing clotting that he referred to as a *thrombotic storm* seen in patients with catastrophic APS. These clots continue to generate thrombin, fibrinolysis is depressed by an increase in plasminogen activator inhibitors ("fibrinolytic shutdown"), and there is simultaneous elevation of coagulation activation products comprising prothrombin activation products F1 and 2, thrombin–antithrombin (TAT) complexes, and protein C activation peptide. There is *also* consumption of the natural anticoagulant proteins such as protein C, protein S, and antithrombin III. That clot removal may indeed be associated with remission of catastrophic APS as evidenced by the report of two patients in whom amputation of gangrenous limbs was associated with complete recovery [17].

Role of complement

The role of complement in aPL-induced thrombosis has received great attention recently [18]. The work on the role of complement in the etiopathogenesis of fetal loss in murine models from the Salmon group in New York [19] has recently been extended by the group from Harvard University in Boston, and might help to explain some of the odd features of the catastrophic APS. Hart and colleagues [20] and Fleming and colleagues [21] demonstrated that complement activation plays an important role not only in local tissue injury but also in remote injury. It is possible that gut barrier dysfunction (eg, from ischemia induced by small vessel occlusive disease in the catastrophic APS) may lead to bacterial translocation to the lung resulting in increased complement neutrophil infiltration as a result of lectin complement pathway activation via ficolins. Mannose-binding lectin activates the lectin complement in the intestines; ficolins may be activating complement in the lungs. This hypothesis explains why, with neutrophilic infiltration initially, secondary disruption of alveolar blood vessels might take place, resulting in diffuse alveolar hemorrhage, a not infrequent accompaniment of the catastrophic APS.

The high frequency of abdominal symptomatology in patients with catastrophic APS and the much higher frequency of pulmonary complications such as alveolar hemorrhage in this group of patients lends circumstantial credence to this link. The hypothesis implicating ficolins also ties in well with the high frequency of infections as "triggering" mechanisms for catastrophic APS.

The work of Hart and colleagues [20] led them to propose a disease model in which aPL could bind to tissues subjected to ischemia/reperfusion insult and mediate tissue damage in the same manner that they mediate fetal growth resorptions when injected into pregnant mice.

Toll-like receptor phenotypic abnormalities

The role of phenotypic abnormalities in toll-like receptors (TLR) (particularly TLR-4)—key functioning proteins present on endothelium, monocytes, and platelets—in patients with catastrophic APS is possibly another important underlying pathogenetic mechanism that is currently being investigated to explain the etiopathogenesis of this unique condition.

International registry

The international registry of patients with catastrophic APS (CAPS Registry) was created in 2000 by the *European Forum on Antiphospholipid Antibodies*. It documents the entire clinical, laboratory, and therapeutic data of all published cases with catastrophic APS, as well as of many additional patients whose data has been fully registered. The sources of information are the personal communications of the physicians who treated these patients and the periodically computer-assisted search (Medline) of published reports to locate all cases of patients with catastrophic APS (keywords: catastrophic, antiphospholipid, catastrophic antiphospholipid syndrome).

This registry can be freely consulted at site (www.med.ub.es/MIMMUN/ FORUM/CAPS.HTM), and it is expected that the periodic analysis of these data will allow us to increase our knowledge of this condition.

Clinical features

Until February 2005, the CAPS Registry included 250 patients: 177 (70.8%) female and 73 (29.2%) male; mean age, 37 ± 14 years; range 7 to 76; 116 (47.5%) with primary APS, 100 (41%) with systemic lupus erythematosus (SLE), 12 (4.7%) with lupus-like syndrome, and 16 with other diseases.

Patients may develop catastrophic APS de novo, without any previous history of a thrombosis either associated with a "primary" APS or SLE. However, it can be seen that previous deep vein thrombosis, fetal loss, or thrombocytopenia are the most frequently encountered aPL-associated previous manifestations.

The clinical manifestations of catastrophic APS mainly depend on two factors: (1) organs affected by the thrombotic event and the extent of the thrombosis, and (2) manifestations of the systemic inflammatory response syndrome (SIRS), which are presumed to be due to excessive cytokine release from affected and necrotic tissues. There are thus two separate and distinct sets of manifestations, each of which requires effective therapy. There are distinct differences between patients with the simple/classic APS and those with the catastrophic APS (Box 1).

Thrombotic manifestations

Intraabdominal thrombotic complications affecting the kidneys, adrenal glands, splenic, intestinal, and mesenteric or pancreatic vasculature are most commonly encountered and the patients frequently present initially with abdominal pain or discomfort. Renal disease is present in 70% of patients but patients do not succumb from uremia (Fig. 1).

Pulmonary complications are next in frequency, with ARDS [22] and pulmonary emboli accounting for the majority, with pulmonary hemorrhage, microthrombi, pulmonary edema, and infiltrates occurring in a minority of patients. Dyspnea is a common presenting symptom.

Skin complications, such as *livedo reticularis*, purpura, and skin necrosis, are next, occurring in 66%.

Cerebral manifestations (infarcts, encephalopathy, seizures, or cerebral venous occlusions) are frequent (60%). Small-vessel cerebrovascular occlusive disease is probably commoner than has been reported, and may be the etiology of the encephalopathic features of the syndrome.

Cardiac problems occur in 53%, with valve defects (mitral, aortic) often present. Myocardial infarctions are a presenting feature in 25% of cases.

Additionally, other organs may be occasionally affected, including testicular/ovarian infarction, necrosis of the prostate, acalculous cholecystitis, bone

---

Box 1. Distinct differences of patients with catastrophic APS

I. Unusual organs affected (eg, ovaries, uterus, testes) with thrombosis of small vessels causing infarctions.

II. High frequency of pulmonary complications such as ARDS or diffuse alveolar hemorrhage.

III. Patients often present with abdominal pain because of intraabdominal vascular complications affecting bowel, gall bladder, pancreas, adrenal glands, spleen.

IV. Early loss of consciousness complicating SIRS.

V. Serologic evidence of disseminated intravascular coagulation without hemorrhagic manifestations in one fifth of patients. This may cause problems in differential diagnosis.

VI. Severe thrombocytopenias, which may result in hemorrhage (particularly cerebral).

VII. High frequency of hemolysis, elevated liver enzymes, and low platelet (HELLP) syndrome in pregnancy-associated cases.

VIII. Poor prognosis.

---

marrow infarction, esophageal rupture, giant gastric ulceration, colonic ulcerations, thrombotic pancreatitis, and adrenal infarction, among other features.

Recurrent catastrophic antiphospholipid syndrome

Recurrences/relapses of the condition are distinctly uncommon and have occurred in less than 10 patients [23–25]. Infections, trauma (eg, minor surgery such as removal of simple cataract), fracture are some of the "triggers" documented, while in others, no specific precipitating factors have been identifiable.

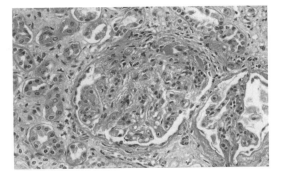

Fig. 1. Renal microangiopathic thrombosis.

Manifestations of the systemic inflammatory response syndrome

This syndrome has been extensively reviewed [26]. Although actual measurements of cytokine levels in very ill patients with catastrophic APS have not been undertaken, it is assumed that this process is ongoing in the acute phase of the illness. Certainly, some of the nonthrombotic manifestations, particularly ARDS [22], are frequently encountered in SIRS. The cytokines involved include tumor necrosis factor (TNF)-α, IL-1, IL-6, and macrophage-migration inhibitory factor, and they are responsible not only for ARDS but also for the cerebral edema that may be a factor in the initial confusion and deterioration of consciousness seen in these patients as well as myocardial dysfunction encountered. IL-18 is also implicated in acute lung inflammation via increasing neutrophil migration and lung vascular permeability, and this cytokine may also be implicated in the pathogenesis of ARDS. This may be superimposed on an underlying infective process, which itself may have been instrumental in "triggering" catastrophic APS. Therefore, in treatment, strong consideration should be given to the early institution of antibiotic therapy.

ARDS associated with septic shock and severe trauma is often complicated by disseminated intravascular coagulation (DIC), a not infrequent finding in patients with catastrophic APS [27].

Laboratory features

Thrombocytopenia is usually present, and was detected in more than 60% of cases from the CAPS Registry. One third have evidence of hemolysis and 20% have some of the features of DIC [20]. Schistocytes, if present, are usually scanty, unlike the abundant numbers seen in patients with TTP [28]. IgG anticardiolipin antibodies (aCL) are usually positive with IgM being less frequent. Patients with SLE demonstrate positive antinuclear antibodies, antibodies to double-stranded DNA and to extractable nuclear antigens (ENA).

Preliminary classification criteria

During the 10th International Congress on aPL in Taormina, Sicily, Italy, in 2002, proposed preliminary classification criteria for the catastrophic APS (Box 2) were accepted in [9]. This consensus statement is of major importance, as patients with a debatable diagnosis or with less severe disease ("probable" catastrophic APS) may now be classified separately and distinctly from those with a "definite" catastrophic APS. These criteria will now provide a more consistent diagnostic paradigm, and will assist in planning and documenting future multicentre studies.

From the analysis of the initial 176 patients included in the CAPS Registry [10], 89 (51%) of the previously compiled patients with catastrophic APS were

---

Box 2. Preliminary criteria for the classification of catastrophic APS

1. Evidence of involvement of three or more organs, systems, or tissues.[a]
2. Development of manifestations simultaneously or in less than a week.
3. Confirmation by histopathology of small vessel occlusion in at least one organ or tissue.[b]
4. Laboratory confirmation of the presence of antiphospholipid antibodies (lupus anticoagulant or anticardiolipin antibodies).[c]

---

[a] Usually, clinical evidence of vessel occlusions, confirmed by imaging techniques when appropriate. Renal involvement is defined by a 50% rise in serum creatinine, severe systemic hypertension (>180/100 mmHg) or proteinuria (>500 mg/24 hours).

[b] For histopathologic confirmation, significant evidence of thrombosis must be present, although vasculitis may coexist occasionally.

[c] If the patient had not been previously diagnosed as having an APS, the laboratory confirmation requires that presence of antiphospholipid antibodies must be detected on two or more occasions at least 6 weeks apart (not necessarily at the time of the event), according to the proposed preliminary criteria for the classification of definite APS [9].

Definite catastrophic APS:
- All four criteria

Probable catastrophic APS:
- All four criteria, except for only two organs, systems, or tissues involvement.
- All four criteria, except for the absence of laboratory confirmation at least 6 weeks apart due to the early death of a patient never previously tested for aPL before the catastrophic APS event.
- 1, 2, and 4
- 1, 3, and 4 and the development of a third event in more than a week but less than a month, despite anticoagulation.

---

classified as having "definite" and 70 (40%) as "probable" catastrophic APS. The sensitivity of these criteria was 90.3% and the specificity 99.4%. Positive and negative predictive values were 99.4% and 91.1%, respectively.

Differential diagnosis

Careful differential diagnosis is mandatory in the presence of a patient with multiorgan thromboses and failure, and this should include catastrophic

APS as well as other microangiopathic syndromes (Table 2), which have overlapping features of (1) thrombotic microangiopathy, (2) hemolytic anemia, (3) thrombocytopenia, and (4) involvement of central nervous and renal systems [28]. These conditions include TTP, hemolytic–uremic syndrome, malignant hypertension, heparin-induced thrombocytopenia, and the HELLP syndrome.

Approximately, one third of patients with catastrophic APS develop serologic or hematologic evidence of DIC during the course of their multiorgan illness [27]. The serologic features of DIC found in these patients may be explicable on the basis of extensive small vessel endothelial damage, such as is also seen accompanying ARDS and SIRS.

The differential diagnosis should also include marantic endocarditis. As many patients have valve lesions as part of their underling SLE or, indeed, primary APS, their presence does not necessarily indicate marantic endocarditis with embolic complications. Cryoglobulinemia, vasculitis, and multiple cholesterol emboli also must be considered.

Treatment

Management of the catastrophic APS is challenging for all attending physicians. Early diagnosis and aggressive therapies are essential to "rescue" such patients from succumbing to this potentially fatal condition. Unfortunately, at this time, despite all therapies advised, the mortality is extremely high (around 50%). An algorithm with treatment guidelines for the catastrophic APS (Fig. 2) has recently been proposed [9]. Treatment may be divided into three major categories: (1) prophylactic therapy, (2) specific therapies, and (3) nonspecific therapies.

Prophylactic therapy

As it is unclear why some patients with APS will develop recurrent episodes and others (a minority) will be "catapulted" into multiorgan failure,

Table 2
Differential diagnosis of thrombotic microangiopathic hemolytic anemia

	HUS	Catastrophic APS	TTP	Malignant hypertension
Thrombocytopenia	+	++	+++	+
Microangiopathic hemolytic anemia	+	+	+	+
Fever	+	+/−	++	−
CNS involvement	+	++	+++	+
Renal involvement	+++	+	+	++
Hypertension	+	+/−	+/−	+++

Abbreviations: APS, antiphospholipid syndrome; CNS, central nervous system; HUS, hemolytic–uremic syndrome; TTP, thrombotic thrombocytopenic purpura.

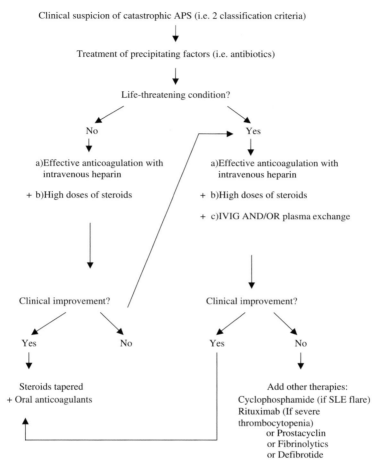

Fig. 2. Treatment of algorith of catastrophic APS.

therefore, in any APS patient particular attention should be given to the following guidelines:

1. Any infection, however trivial, should be energetically treated with the appropriate antibiotics.
2. APS patients undergoing surgical procedures, however minor, should all receive parenteral anticoagulation during the procedure instead of remaining on coumadin.
3. The puerperium should be adequately covered for a minimum of 6 weeks with parenteral anticoagulants (eg, subcutaneous heparin).
4. SLE "flares," although uncommonly associated with catastrophic APS, should also be treated with parenteral anticoagulation.

Specific therapies

First-line therapies
Intravenous heparin. Intravenous heparin (1500 U/h) is usually administered for 7 to 10 days followed by oral anticoagulants to an international normalized ratio of approximately 3.

Corticosteroids. Corticosteriods (1–2 mg/kg/day) should be administered for a minimum of 3 days, but may have to be continued for longer depending on the patient's response. Steroids are not indicated for the treatment of the ongoing thrombosis or to attempt to reduce the high levels of aPL, but to treat the manifestations of the presumed excessive cytokine release because of the widespread tissue necrosis. ARDS is a prime example of this.

Second-line therapies
Intravenous immunoglobulins. The daily dose recommended for intravenous immunoglobulins (IVIGs) is 0.4 g/d/kg body weight for 4 to 5 days. It may specifically be helpful in those patients who have severe thrombocytopenia, but also possibly decreases antibody synthesis and increases the catabolism of circulating immunoglobulins in others. There is no evidence, judging from the analysis of treated patients with catastrophic APS, that IVIGs on its own improves survival, but its combination with plasma exchange might be more effective. IVIGs are usually well tolerated, but there are a few reports of thromboembolic events after IVIG infusions, and a few cases have been described on the association of acute renal failure with IVIG therapy.

Plasma exchange. Pathogenic IgG aCL and β2-GPI as well as cytokines such as IL-I, IL-6, TNF-α, and complement may be removed by this procedure. It has been reported as improving the outcome in patients with catastrophic APS and, of course, is the treatment of choice in patients with features of microangiopathic hemolytic anemia where the emphasis is on small vessel occlusive disease.

Third-line therapies
    These comprise several compounds that have either been used fairly often (cyclophosphamide) or in a few cases only (rituximab, prostacyclines, ancrod, defibrotide), and may have contributed to the recovery of the patient.

Cyclosphosphamide. Theoretically, immunosuppressive therapy might be useful to prevent rebound of the aPL following plasma exchange.

Rituximab. This anti-CD20 monoclonal antibody has now been used with good results in patients with nonresponsive severe thrombocytopenia [29].

Prostacyclin. This compound is a potent inhibitor of platelet aggregation, and would thus theoretically be of benefit in the ongoing clotting process. It is also a vasodilator. The dose is 5 ng/kg/min for 7 days.

CATASTROPHIC ANTIPHOSPHOLIPID SYNDROME

Ancrod. It is a powerful fibrinolytic, and also corrects plasminogen activator deficiencies. It is seldom used today.

Defibrotide. This is an alkali metal salt of single-stranded DNA, and has antithrombotic properties. Because of its polypharmacologic properties, indications are that it may have an important role to play in the future in the management of refractory patients with catastrophic APS and has been successfully used in one patient.

Other fibrinolytics (eg, streptokinase, urokinase, tissue plasminogen activators). These compounds, theoretically, might have an important role to play in the management of refractory patients with catastrophic APS but may be associated with hemorrhagic complications. Their judicious use in these difficult cases where a life-threatening situation is imminent because of ongoing clotting is probably justified.

Nonspecific therapies

Most patients end up in ICU because multiorgan failure has supervened. If renal failure is present, hemodialysis may be required. Mechanical ventilation for respiratory failure is often indicated, particularly if ARDS is present. Inotropic drugs for circulatory failure need to be administered. Severe hypertension due to renal vascular occlusive disease may necessitate aggressive antihypertensive therapy. If hypotension is present due either to myocardial depression (SIRS), microangiopathy of small cardiac vessels or hemorrhagic infarction of the adrenal glands, parenteral steroids are necessary. This is another reason for inotropic drugs.

Outcome and prognosis

The mortality of the condition is high despite present-day therapy. Mortality is of the order of 50%. In a recent analysis of the CAPS Registry focused on mortality [30], the major cause of death was identified in 81 of 114 (71.1%) patients. Cerebral involvement was the most frequent cause of death, being present in 22 patients (27.2%). They included stroke in 15 (18.5%), cerebral hemorrhage in 4 (4.9%), and encephalopathy in 3 (3.7%) patients. Cardiac involvement was identified in 16 (19.8%) patients as major cause of death, including cardiac failure in 14 (17.3%) and arrhythmias in 2 (2.5%) patients. Infection was described as the main cause of death in 16 (19.8%) patients, including bacterial sepsis in 10 (12.3%), fungal sepsis in 3 (3.7%), *Pneumocystis carinii* pneumonia in 2 (2.5%) patients, and suppurative peritonitis in 1 patient (1.2%). Multiorgan failure was identified in 14 (17.3%) patients. Pulmonary involvement was presented as major cause of death in eight (9.8%) patients, mainly consisting of ARDS in six (7.4%), and pulmonary embolism and pulmonary hemorrhage (one case each). Abdominal involvement was incriminated as main cause of death in four

(4.9%) patients, including liver failure in three (3.7%) and acute abdomen in one (1.2%), respectively.

Necropsy was performed in 58 of 114 (50.8%) patients. The main occlusive features were microthrombosis, present in 49 (84.5%) patients, followed by infarcts in 31 (53.4%), thromboses of large vessels in 11 (18.9%), and pulmonary embolism in 7 (12.1%). In order of frequency, the kidneys (65.3%), the heart (55.1%), the lungs (48.9%), the brain (48.9%), the spleen (24.5%), the skin (22.4%), the gut (20.4%), the liver (20.4%), and the adrenal glands (16.3%) were the main organs affected by microthromboses. Other organs where microthromboses were occasionally described included pancreas, uterus, testicles, retina, bone marrow, thyroid, muscles, and peripheral nerves.

However, once patients with catastrophic APS have recovered, patients usually have a stable course with continued anticoagulation. A recent paper [31] has documented that 66% of patients with catastrophic APS who have survived the initial event had remained symptom free for an average follow-up of 62.7 months. Twenty-six percent of the survivors, however, developed further APS-related events. Only few patients have suffered "recurrent" catastrophic APS [23–25]. In these, clear precipitating factors were evident, for example, recurrent infections and trauma. This is a rare event, unlike patients with the not superficially dissimilar condition of TTP where recurrent episodes are common.

Summary

Catastrophic APS is a potentially life-threatening condition with a high mortality, which requires high clinical awareness. New mechanisms for its production can only be explored if samples are obtained, stored, and dispatched to investigation sites in Europe (Barcelona), the United States (Atlanta), and Japan (Sapporo). Details will be posted and made available on the International Registry Web Site in 2006. It is essential that the condition be diagnosed early and treated aggressively. The combination of high doses of iv heparin, iv steroids plus repeated doses of iv gammaglobulins or plasma exchange is the treatment of choice in patients with this severe condition. Additionally, preventive measures in patients with APS may be effective if the development of the catastrophic APS is to be avoided.

References

[1] Asherson RA. The catastrophic antiphospholipid antibody syndrome. J Rheumatol 1992;
    19:508–12.
[2] Piette JC, Cervera R, Levy R, et al. The catastrophic antiphospholipid syndrome—Asherson's syndrome. Ann Med Intern 2003;154:95–6.
[3] Greisman SG, Thayaparan R-S, Godwin TA, et al. Occlusive vasculopathy in systemic lupus erythematosus—association with anticardiolipin antibody. Arch Intern Med 1991;151:
    389–92.

[4] Harris EN, Bos K. An acute disseminated coagulopathy-vasculopathy associated with the antiphopholipid syndrome. Arch Intern Med 1991;151:231–2.

[5] Asherson RA, Cervera R, Piette JC, et al. Catastrophic antiphospholipid syndrome. Clinical and laboratory features of 50 patients. Medicine (Baltimore) 1998;77:195–207.

[6] Asherson RA, Cervera R, Piette JC, et al. Catastrophic antiphospholipid syndrome: clues to the pathogenesis from a series of 80 patients. Medicine (Baltimore) 2001;80:355–76.

[7] Cervera R, Piette JC, Font J, et al. Antiphospholipid syndrome: clinical and immunologic manifestations and patterns of disease expression in a cohort of 1,000 patients. Arthritis Rheum 2002;46:1019–27.

[8] Cervera R, Font J, Tincani A, et al. V Meeting of the European Forum on Antiphospholipid Antibodies. Autoimmun Rev, in press.

[9] Asherson RA, Cervera R, de Groot P, et al. Catastrophic antiphospholipid syndrome: international consensus statement on classification criteria and treatment guidelines. Lupus 2003; 12:530–4.

[10] Cervera R, Font J, Gómez-Puerta JA, et al. Validation of the preliminary criteria for the classification of catastrophic antiphospholipid syndrome. Ann Rheum Dis 2005;64: 1205–9.

[11] Asherson RA, Shoenfeld Y. The role of infection in the pathogenesis of catastrophic antiphospholipid syndrome—molecular mimicry? J Rheumatol 2000;27:12–4.

[12] Gharavi E, Cucurull E, Tang H, et al. Induction of antiphospholipid antibodies by immunization with viral peptides. Lupus 1999;8:449–55.

[13] Gharavi AE, Pierangeli SS, Harris N. New developments in viral peptides and antiphospholipid antibody induction. J Autoimmun 2000;15:227–30.

[14] Shoenfeld Y, Blank M, Cervera R, et al. Infectious origin of the antiphospholipid syndrome. Ann Rheum Dis 2006;65:2–6.

[15] Gómez-Puerta JA, Cervera R, Espinosa G, et al. Antiphospholipid antibodies associated with malignancies: clinical and pathological characteristics of 120 patients. Semin Arthritis Rheum 2006;35:322–32.

[16] Kitchens CS. Thrombotic storm: when thrombosis begets thrombosis. Am J Med 1998;104: 381–5.

[17] Amital H, Levy Y, Davidson C, et al. Catastrophic antiphospholipid syndrome: remission following leg amputation. Semin Arthritis Rheum 2001;31:127–32.

[18] Pierangeli SS, Girardi G, Vega-Ostertag M, et al. Requirement of activation of complement C3 and C5 for antiphospholipid antibody mediated thrombosis. Arthritis Rheum 2005;52: 2120–4.

[19] Salmon JE, Girardi G, Holers VM. Activation of complement mediates antiphospholipid antibody–induced pregnancy loss. Lupus 2003;12:535–8.

[20] Hart ML, Keonzo KA, Shaffer LA, et al. Gastrointestinal ischemia—reperfusion is lectin complement pathway dependent without involving C1q. J Immunol 2005;174:6373–80.

[21] Fleming SD, Egan RE, Chai C, et al. Anti-phospholipid antibodies restore mesenteric ischemia reperfusion-induced injury in complement receptor 2/complement receptor 1-deficient mice. J Immunol 2005;173:7055–61.

[22] Bucciarelli S, Espinosa G, Asherson RA, et al. The acute respiratory distress syndrome in catastrophic antiphospholipid syndrome: analysis of a series of 47 patients. Ann Rheum Dis 2006;65:81–6.

[23] Undas A, Swadzba J, Undas R, et al. Three episodes of acute multiorgan failure in a woman with secondary antiphospholipid syndrome. Pol Arch Med Wewn 1998;100:556–60.

[24] Cerveny KC, Sawitzke AD. Relapsing catastrophic antiphospholipid antibody syndrome: a mimic for thrombotic thrombocytopenic purpura? Lupus 1999;8:477–81.

[25] Gordon A, McLean CA, Ryan P, et al. Steroid-responsive catastrophic antiphospholipid syndrome. J Gastroenterol Hepatol 2004;19:479–80.

[26] Belmont HM, Abramson SB, Lie JT. Pathology and pathogenesis of vascular injury in systemic lupus erythematosus. Arthritis Rheum 1996;39:9–22.

[27] Asherson RA, Espinosa G, Cervera R, et al. Disseminated intravascular coagulation in catastrophic antiphospholipid syndrome: clinical and haematological characteristics of 23 patients. Ann Rheum Dis 2005;64:943–6.

[28] Espinosa G, Bucciarelli S, Cervera R, et al. Thrombotic microangiopathic haemolytic anaemia and antiphospholipid antibodies. Ann Rheum Dis 2004;63:730–6.

[29] Ehresmann S, Arkfeld D, Shinada S, et al. A novel therapeutic approach for catastrophic antiphospholipid syndrome (CAPS) when conventional therapy with anticoagulants and steroids were unsuccessful. Ann Rheum Dis 2004;64(Suppl): FR10278 (abstr.) 70.

[30] Bucciarelli S, Espinosa G, Cervera R, et al. Mortality in the catastrophic antiphospholipid syndrome: Causes of death and prognostic factors in a series of 250 patients. Arthritis Rheum, in press.

[31] Erkan D, Asherson RA, Espinosa G, et al. The long-term outcome of catastrophic antiphospholipid syndrome survivors. Ann Rheum Dis 2003;62:530–3.

ELSEVIER
SAUNDERS

Rheum Dis Clin N Am
32 (2006) 591–607

RHEUMATIC
DISEASE CLINICS
OF NORTH AMERICA

Management of Antiphospholipid Syndrome in Pregnancy

Michelle Petri, MD, MPH*, Umair Qazi, MD, MPH

Department of Medicine, Division of Rheumatology, Johns Hopkins University School of Medicine, 1830 E. Monument 7500, East Baltimore Campus, Baltimore, MD 21205, USA

Antiphospholipid antibody syndrome is one of the most important acquired causes of hypercoagulability and pregnancy loss [1]. Antiphospholipoid syndrome (APS) patients are prone to arterial as well as venous thrombosis [2]. Pregnancy itself is a procoagulant state, to compensate for excessive maternal bleeding during delivery. In addition, venous stasis due to venous dilation and compression of the uterus [3] occurs, leading also to a higher risk of thrombosis. The goal of treatment of APS in pregnancy is to protect the mother from thrombosis and to reduce the risk of fetal loss. This article will review current treatment options for antiphospholipid antibodies in pregnancy.

Pathogenesis

Understanding of the pathogenesis of pregnancy loss in APS would ultimately lead to scientifically derived, rather than empiric, therapy. The most important advance in this area has been in a murine model of APS pregnancy loss. In this model, complement activation is a necessary step, and blocking complement activation or complement deficiency is protective [4]. At least in the mouse, this work suggests that complement activation, and not thrombosis, is the pathogenetic mechanism of APS pregnancy loss. This has been further confirmed by studies of different anticoagulants. Levels of heparin, which block complement activation but do not achieve anticoagulation, are able to protect against APS pregnancy loss [5]. A national multicenter study is now underway, called PROMISSE, to determine

* Corresponding author.
E-mail address: mpetri@jhmi.edu (M. Petri).

0889-857X/06/$ - see front matter © 2006 Elsevier Inc. All rights reserved.
doi:10.1016/j.rdc.2006.05.007   *rheumatic.theclinics.com*

if complement activation precedes pregnancy loss in pregnant women with antiphospholipid antibodies versus pregnant controls.

If complement activation proves to be the major mechanism of pregnancy loss in women with APS, it would have implications for treatment. First, it would suggest that prophylactic doses of heparin would be effective (without aspirin). Second, it would suggest that prednisone might have a role, after decades in which prednisone has been discouraged because of its maternal morbidity, and, especially, its role in increasing pre-eclampsia. Finally, specific blockade of complement activation could be on the research horizon, through monoclonal antibodies or other inhibitory techniques.

Before the work on complement activation shook the field, a large body of work already existed on effects of antiphospholipid antibodies that could be injurious to pregnancy. Early pregnancy loss is still poorly understood. Antiphospholipid antibodies may affect implantation [6]. Interleukin 3, for example, may be important in early pregnancy loss, and might be one of the benefits of aspirin therapy [7]. Antiphospholipid antibodies could lead to later pregnancy loss through multiple mechanisms of injury to the uteroplacental unit, including interfering with annexin V [8].

Evidence-based management

Clinical trials of treatment of APS pregnancy suffer from common weaknesses. First, there is not a uniform definition of early pregnancy losses, nor stratification by history of early versus late losses. Second, there is not a stratification by anticardiolipin versus lupus anticoagulant positivity, nor proof of persistence of antiphospholipid antibodies. Third, there is no agreement on whether treatments should be started pre- or postconception, or whether some should be stopped before delivery.

Clinical trials of aspirin

Many APS pregnancy trials have included aspirin (Table 1). However, many have included aspirin in both arms of the trial, so that no conclusion regarding the benefit (or harm) of aspirin alone can be ascertained. Several trials, however, contained an "aspirin alone" arm.

Aspirin has been compared with placebo in several APS pregnancy trials. Tulppala and colleagues [9] compared aspirin 50 mg daily versus placebo in 66 women. Only 12 had antiphospholipid antibodies, however. Aspirin had no benefit over placebo. Cowchock and colleagues [10] compared aspirin 81 mg daily versus usual care in 19 pregnancies. Aspirin had no advantage. Pattison and all [11] compared aspirin 75 mg daily versus placebo in 50 pregnancies. No difference was found in either antenatal or neonatal morbidity.

Kutteh, in 1996 [12], compared aspirin 81 mg as a sole therapy versus aspirin plus unfractionated heparin. The aspirin was started preconception. Heparin was started at 10,000 units subcutaneously in two divided doses,

Table 1
APS pregnancy trials including aspirin

Author	Year	Size	Study design	Comparison arm 1	Comparison arm 2	Study outcome
Cowchock [15]	1992	45	Randomized multicenter	Prednisone 20 mg Aspirin 80 mg	Heparin 10,000 units twice daily Aspirin 80 mg	No difference (75% live births) in pregnancy success. More maternal morbidity and preterm delivery with prednisone/aspirin
Silver [30]	1993	34	Randomized	Aspirin 81 mg	Prednisone 20 mg with subsequent adjustment based on anticardiolipin level Aspirin 81 mg	No difference in pregnancy success (100%). Preterm delivery was higher with prednisone/aspirin ($P = 0.003$).
Kutteh [44]	1996	50	Prospective unicenter Consecutive assignment	Aspirin 81 mg High-dose heparin	Aspirin 81 mg Low-dose heparin	No difference
Kutteh [12]	1996	50	Prospective unicenter	Heparin initiated at 10,000 units daily in two divided doses Aspirin 81 mg/d	Aspirin 81 mg	Heparin/aspirin was better
Rai [13]	1997	90	Randomized	UF Heparin 5000 units twice daily Aspirin 75 mg	Aspirin 75 mg	Aspirin/Heparin had better pregnancy outcome as compared to aspirin alone
Tulppala [9]	1997	66 (only 12 had anticardiolipin)	Placebo controlled randomized.	Aspirin 50 mg	Placebo	No difference
Cowchock [10]	1997	19	Randomized	Aspirin 81 mg	Usual care	No difference

(continued on next page)

Table 1 (*continued*)

Author	Year	Size	Study design	Comparison arm 1	Comparison arm 2	Study outcome
Branch [27]	2000	16	Randomized	Aspirin 81 mg Heparin 15,000–20,000 units	Aspirin 81 mg Heparin 15,000–20,000 units IVIG 1 g/kg for 2 consecutive days every 4 weeks	No difference
Pattison [11]	2000	50	Randomized placebo controlled	Aspirin 75 mg	Placebo	No difference: 85% pregnancy success in placebo versus 80% with aspirin
Pauzner [25]	2001	57	Observational	Enoxaparin Aspirin	Warfarin between weeks 15 to 34	No difference: 86% successful pregnancy with warfarin vs 87% in nonwarfarin
Farquharson [14]	2002	98	Randomized placebo controlled	LMW Heparin 5000 units Aspirin 75 mg	Aspirin 75 mg	No difference
Stephenson [23]	2004	28	Randomized	LMW Heparin Aspirin	Unfractionated Heparin Aspirin	No difference
Jeremic [28]	2005	40	Observational	LMW Heparin Aspirin	LMW Heparin Aspirin Intravenous immunoglobulin	No difference: successful pregnancy in 85% heparin/aspirin and 90% heparin/ aspirin/IVIG

Abbreviations: IVIO, intravenous immunoglobulins; LMW, low molecular weight; UF, unfractionated.

and was adjusted to keep the activated partial thromboplastin times (aPTT) at 1.2 to 1.5. This was a one center trial, with 50 women. The heparin and aspirin group did better than the aspirin alone group. Similarly, Rai and colleagues, in 1997 [13], compared aspirin 75 mg as a sole therapy with unfractionated heparin 5000 units subcutaneously twice daily with aspirin. The aspirin was begun after a positive pregnancy test. Heparin was started at the time a fetal heart beat was demonstrated on ultrasound. Ninety women were randomized. As with the Kutteh trial, the heparin and aspirin group did better than the aspirin-alone group. The very similar results from these two trials suggest that heparin dosing does not need to be adjusted for any certain aPPT.

A third trial, done by Farquharson and colleagues, that compared aspirin alone versus heparin and aspirin, reached a different conclusion from Kutteh and Rai and colleagues [14]. Aspirin 75 mg daily as a sole therapy was compared with aspirin 75 mg plus low molecular weight (LWM) heparin 5000 units subcutaneously daily. Ninety-eight women participated in this randomized placebo-controlled trial. In this study, aspirin and heparin/aspirin were equal in successful pregnancies.

Clinical trials of heparin

Heparin has been studied in multiple APS pregnancy trials (Table 2). One of the most pivotal clinical trials compared prednisone and aspirin with unfractionated heparin and aspirin [15]. In this multicenter trial, both arms had equal pregnancy success. Maternal morbidity, however, including gestational diabetes and preterm birth, due largely to pre-eclampsia, was increased in the prednisone/aspirin arm. This trial had immediate impact on clinical obstetric practice, with heparin/aspirin becoming the "gold standard" treatment.

Subsequent trials (also reviewed under "Clinical Trials of Aspirin") compared whether heparin added benefit over aspirin alone (Table 3). These three clinical trials, Kutteh [12], Rai and colleagues [13], and Farquharson and colleagues [14] reached different conclusions, with Kutteh and Rai and colleagues finding superiority of heparin/aspirin and Farquharson and colleagues finding no difference. There were design differences between the trials. Both Kutteh and Rai and colleagues used unfractionated heparin, whereas Farquharson and colleagues used LMW heparin. Kutteh started aspirin before conception, whereas Rai and Farquharson and colleagues started it after conception. Kutteh adjusted the heparin dose. Rai and colleagues started heparin after the finding of a fetal heart beat on fetal ultrasound. However, none of these design differences appears to explain the contrasting results.

LMW heparin may offer an advantage over unfractionated heparin in terms of convenience, less osteoporosis [16–18], and less thrombocytopenia [19,20]. There is disagreement over whether LMW heparin can or should be

Table 2
APS pregnancy trials including heparin

Author	Year	Size	Study design	Comparison arm 1	Comparison arm 2	Study outcome
Cowchock [15]	1992	45	Randomized multicenter	Prednisone 20 mg Aspirin 80 mg	Heparin 10,000 units twice daily Aspirin 80 mg	No difference (75% live births) in pregnancy success. More maternal morbidity and preterm delivery with prednisone/aspirin
Kutteh [12]	1996	50	Prospective unicenter	Heparin initiated at 10,000 units daily in two divided doses Aspirin 81 mg	Aspirin 81 mg	Heparin/aspirin was better
Rai [13]	1997	90	Randomized	UF Heparin 5000 units twice daily Aspirin 75 mg	Aspirin 75 mg	Heparin/aspirin had better pregnancy outcome as compared to aspirin alone
Branch [27]	2000	16	Randomized Trial	Aspirin 81 mg Heparin 15,000–20,000 units	Aspirin 81 mg Heparin 15,000–20,000 units IVIG 1g/kg for 2 consecutive days every 4 weeks	No difference
Pauzner [25]	2001	57	Observational	Enoxaparin Aspirin	Warfarin between weeks 15 to 34	No difference: 86% successful pregnancy with warfarin versus 87% in non-warfarin
Farquharson [14]	2002	98	Randomized placebo Controlled	LMW Heparin 5000 units Aspirin 75 mg	Aspirin 75 mg	No difference
Triolo [45]	2003	40	Randomized	LMW Heparin 5700 units Aspirin 75 mg	IVIG 400 mg/kg/d for 2 days then once every month	IVIG was inferior (57% successful pregnancies vs 84% with heparin/aspirin)

Study	Year	N	Study type	Treatment	Comparison	Outcome
Malinowski [46]	2003	148	Randomized	Aspirin 75 mg	LMW Heparin Group 3: LMW Heparin Aspirin 75 mg	No difference: aspirin (89.3%), heparin (81.1%), aspirin/heparin (92.5%) Pregnancy loss was statistically higher in the lupus anticoagulant group (21.2%) versus anticardiolipin (6.7%)
Ensom [22]	2004	15	Pharmacokinetic randomized study	Various doses of dalteparin	Various doses of UF Heparin	Dalteparin dosing requires adjustment during pregnancy: 2500 units daily pre- and postpregnancy; 5000 units daily in pregnancy
Stephenson [23]	2004	28	Randomized	LMW Heparin Aspirin	Unfractionated Heparin Aspirin	No difference
Jeremic [28]	2005	40	Observational	LMW Heparin Aspirin	LMW Heparin Aspirin Intravenous immunoglobulin	No difference: successful pregnancy in 85% heparin/aspirin and 90% heparin/aspirin/IVIG
Noble [24]	2005	50	Randomized	LMW heparin Aspirin	UF heparin Aspirin	No difference: 84% live birth with LMWH vs 80% with UF heparin

Abbreviations: IVIO, intravenous immunoglobulins; LMW, low molecular weight; UF, unfractionated.

Table 3
Comparison of heparin/aspirin versus aspirin for APS pregnancies

Author	Year	Size	Study design	Comparison arm 1	Comparison arm 2	Study outcome
Kutteh [12]	1996	50	Prospective unicenter	Heparin initiated at 10,000 units daily in two divided doses Aspirin 81 mg/d	Aspirin 81 mg	Heparin/aspirin was better
Rai [13]	1997	90	Randomized	UF Heparin 5000 units twice daily Aspirin 75 mg	Aspirin 75 mg	Heparin/aspirin had better pregnancy outcome as compared to aspirin alone
Farquharson [14]	2002	98	Randomized Placebo Controlled	LMW Heparin 5000 units Aspirin 75 mg	Aspirin 75 mg	No difference

Abbreviations: IVIO, intravenous immunoglobulins; LMW, low molecular weight; UF, unfractionated.

used as once daily dosing when being given in prophylactic or therapeutic doses for APS pregnancy. Many units, including our own, believe that twice daily dosing is preferable [21]. One randomized study of pharmacokinetics determined that dalteparin required one dose pre- and postpregnancy and another dose during pregnancy [22].

Two clinical trials have compared unfractionated heparin versus LWM heparin in terms of APS pregnancy efficacy. Stephenson and colleagues compared LMW heparin/aspirin with unfractionated heparin/aspirin in 28 pregnancies and found 69% live births with LMW heparin/aspirin versus 31% with UF heparin/aspirin (not statistically different) [23]. In a second trial, Noble and colleagues found 84% live births with LMW heparin/aspirin versus 80% with unfractionated heparin/aspirin, with 25 pregnancies in each arm [24].

Clinical trials of warfarin

In the United States, because of concern about warfarin teratogenicity, pregnant women are switched to heparin. However, in other countries, warfarin is used, sometimes throughout pregnancy and sometimes after organogenesis. Pauzner and colleagues [25] (Table 4) compared enoxaparin versus warfarin in an observational study in 57 pregnancies and found no difference in outcome.

Clinical trials of intravenous immunoglobulin

In most APS pregnancy trials, only 75% to 80% pregnancy success is obtained, regardless of treatment arm. Women with failed pregnancies on standard treatments such as heparin and aspirin need additional options. Intravenous immunoglobulin (IVIG) is of interest because it reduces levels of anticardiolipin. One mechanism is that saturation of the IgG transport receptor leads to accelerated catabolism of pathogenic antiphospholipid antibodies [26].

IVIG has been studied in three APS pregnancy trials (Table 5). In comparison to LMW heparin and aspirin, IVIG is inferior. In two trials [27,28],

Table 4
APS pregnancy trials including warfarin

Author	Year	Size	Study design	Comparison arm 1	Comparison arm 2	Study outcome
Pauzner [25]	2001	57	Observational	Enoxaparin Low-dose aspirin	Warfarin between weeks 15 to 34	No difference: 86% successful pregnancy with warfarin versus 87% in non-warfarin

Table 5
APS pregnancy trials including intravenous immunoglobulin

Author	Year	Size	Study design	Comparison arm 1	Comparison arm 2	Study outcome
Branch [27]	2000	16	Randomized	Aspirin 81 mg Heparin 15,000–20,000 units	Aspirin 81 mg Heparin 15,000–20,000 units IVIG 1g/kg for 2 consecutive days every 4 weeks	No difference
Triolo [45]	2003	40	Randomized	LMW Heparin 5700 units Aspirin 75 mg	IVIG 400 mg/kg/d for 2 days then once every month	IVIG was inferior (57% successful pregnancies vs 84% with heparin/aspirin)
Jeremic [28]	2005	40	Observational	LMW Heparin Aspirin	LMW Heparin Aspirin Intravenous immunoglobulin	No difference: successful pregnancy in 85% heparin/aspirin and 90% heparin/aspirin/IVIG

Abbreviations: IVIG, intravenous immunoglobulins; LMW, low molecular weight; UF, unfractionated.

IVIG offered no advantage over heparin and aspirin. Given the expense of IVIG, the lack of positive clinical trials suggests it should be reserved for accepted indications in pregnancy, such as thrombocytopenia.

Clinical trials of prednisone

Prednisone was the original APS pregnancy therapy studied by Lubbe [29]. In the landmark trial of Cowchock and colleagues, however, the prednisone/aspirin arm had more maternal morbidity in terms of diabetes mellitus and pre-eclampsia [15]. Subsequently, Silver and colleagues showed that prednisone/aspirin led to more preterm birth [30]. Finally, Laskin and colleagues [31], in a study of 202 pregnancies (not all of which were antiphospholipid antibody positive), determined that prednisone/aspirin was inferior to placebo in terms of preterm birth (Table 6).

Management

Management is summarized in Table 7.

Antiphospholipid antibody positivity with a history of thrombosis but no pregnancy loss

Patients with antiphospholipid antibodies and a first episode of thrombosis have a high rate of recurrent thrombosis [3,32,33]. The Swedish Duration of Anticoagulation Study found an increased mortality as well [34]. For this reason, APS thrombosis is treated with long-term anticoagulation. The targeted degree of anticoagulation has changed, however. Initially, the targeted international normalized ratio (INR) was 3 to 4 ("high intensity"), based on the largest retrospective study [3]. Subsequently, two randomized clinical trials [35,36] have demonstrated that an INR target of 2 to 3 is equally effective as the more dangerous 3 to 4 target.

However, warfarin can be teratogenic in pregnancy. Therefore, as soon as pregnancy is identified, the warfarin is stopped and therapeutic doses of heparin are substituted.

Antiphospholipid antibody positivity and no prior pregnancies

As many as 7.5% of normal controls have antiphospholipid antibodies [37]. On occasion, antiphospholipid antibodies may have been checked and found to be abnormal in a woman with no prior pregnancies nor thrombosis. Possible scenarios include a woman with lupus, a woman with infertility, or a woman with a strong family history of lupus or APS.

If the woman has lupus, and is on hydroxychloroquine for systemic lupus erythematosus (SLE) disease activity, there is a general consensus that hydroxychloroquine can be continued during pregnancy. Although hydroxychloroquine does cross the placenta, and there is the potential for

Table 6
APS pregnancy trials including prednisone

Author	Year	Size	Study design	Comparison arm 1	Comparison arm 2	Study outcome
Cowchock [15]	1992	45	Randomized multicenter	Prednisone 20 mg Aspirin 80 mg	Heparin 10,000 units twice daily Aspirin 80 mg	No difference (75% live births) in pregnancy success. More maternal morbidity and preterm delivery with prednisone/aspirin
Silver [30]	1993	34	Randomized	Aspirin 81 mg	Prednisone 20 mg with subsequent adjustment based on anticardiolipin level Aspirin 81 mg	No difference in pregnancy success (100%). Preterm delivery was higher with prednisone/aspirin ($P = 0.003$).
Laskin [31]	1997	202	Randomized placebo controlled (not all had anticardiolipin or lupus anticoagulant)	Prednisone (0.5 to 0.8 mg/kg) Aspirin 100 mg	Placebo	No difference in pregnancy success (65% with prednisone/aspirin vs 57% placebo). Preterm births were increased with prednisone/aspirin (62% versus 12%, $p < 0.001$), as were hypertension ($p = 0.05$) and diabetes mellitus ($p = 0.02$)

Table 7
Current treatment recommendations for APS pregnancy

Condition	Pregnancy	Postpregnancy
Women with previous thrombosis	Unfractionated or LMW Heparin in therapeutic range	Return to warfarin
Women with antiphospholipid antibodies but no history of pregnancy loss or thromboembolism.	Low dose aspirin	Low-dose aspirin
Women with medium to high titer anticardiolipin, anti-beta2glycoprotein 1, or lupus anticoagulant, and 2–3 (or more) first trimester losses or one or more fetal deaths or one or more very preterm births due to placental insufficiency	Low dose aspirin AND Prophylactic unfractionated or LMW heparin	Continue unfractionated or low molecular weight heparin for 6 weeks postpartum Continue low-dose aspirin life-long

Abbreviations: IVIO, intravenous immunoglobulins; LMW, low molecular weight; UF, unfractionated.

deposition in the fetal eye or ear, a large published experience has not found problems in children exposed in utero [38–40]. Hydroxychloroquine reverses platelet activation induced by human IgG anticardiolipin [41] and reduces thrombosis size in an animal model [42]. If the woman has lupus, low-dose aspirin would be added.

If the woman does not have lupus, most physicians would start low dose aspirin (81 mg), not just during the pregnancy, but as a life-long prophylactic treatment to reduce the risk of future thrombosis. It is important to acknowledge, however, that aspirin has yet to be proven effective as a prophylactic therapy for APS thrombosis. In fact, the randomized prospective clinical trial of Doruk Erkan and colleagues [43] has not shown benefit, although the trial is still ongoing.

Antiphospholipid antibody positivity and one first trimester loss

Although not specifically addressed in clinical trials, the fact that first trimester losses are commonly found in normal women means that first trimester pregnancy loss cannot always be ascribed causally to APS. Thus, most would only recommend low dose aspirin.

Antiphospholipid antibody positivity and multiple first trimester losses or one late fetal loss

The predominance of clinical trial evidence supports the use of prophylactic doses of heparin and aspirin. LMW heparin is equally effective as unfractionated heparin. Twice-daily versus once-daily dosing has not been adequately studied.

Summary

APS pregnancy losses are one of the most common treatable causes of recurrent pregnancy loss. Clinical trials have helped in delineating the dangers of prednisone use in pregnancy, and suggest that heparin and aspirin regimens are preferred. However, the clinical trials suffer from the lack of uniform definition of antiphospholipid antibody positivity, from inclusion of women with different past pregnancy histories, and from different timing of the onset of the therapeutic modalities tested. New research on the role of complement activation in murine APS pregnancy loss may change therapeutic options in the future.

Acknowledgments

The Lupus Cohort was supported by NIAMS R01 #AR43737 and the Johns Hopkins University General Clinical Research Center M01-RR00052. This work was supported by the Kirkland Scholar Program.

References

[1] Petri M. Pathogenesis and treatment of the antiphospholipid antibody syndrome. Med Clin North Am 1997;81:151–78.

[2] Ruiz-Irastorza G, Khamashta MA, Hughes GR. Hughes syndrome crosses boundaries. Autoimmun Rev 2002;1:43–8.

[3] Khamashta MA, Cuadrado MJ, Mujic F, et al. The management of thrombosis in the anti-phospholipid antibody syndrome. N Engl J Med 1995;332:993–7.

[4] Holers VM, Girardi G, Mo L, et al. Complement C3 activation is required for antiphospho-lipid antibody-induced fetal loss. J Exp Med 2002;195(2):211–20.

[5] Girardi G, Redecha P, Salmon JE. Heparin prevents antiphospholipid antibody-induced fe-tal loss by inhibiting complement activation. Nat Med 2004;10(11):1222–6.

[6] Di Simone N, Meroni PL, de Papa N, et al. Antiphospholipid antibodies affect trophoblast gonadotropin secretion and invasiveness by binding directly and through adhered beta2-glycoprotein I. Arthritis Rheum 2000;43(1):140–50.

[7] Shoenfeld Y, Sherer Y, Fishman P. Interleukin-3 and pregnancy loss in antiphospholipid syndrome. Scand J Rheumatol Suppl 1998;107:19–22.

[8] Rand JH, Wu XX, Andree HAM, et al. Pregnancy loss in the antiphospholipid-antibody syndrome—a possible thrombogenic mechanism. N Engl J Med 1997;337(3):154–60.

[9] Tulppala M, Marttunen M, Soderstrom-Anttila V, et al. Low-dose aspirin in prevention of miscarriage in women with unexplained or autoimmune related recurrent miscarriage: effect on prostacyclin and thromboxane A2 production. Hum Reprod 1997;12(7): 1567–72.

[10] Cowchock S, Reece EA. Do low-risk pregnant women with antiphospholipid antibodies need to be treated? Organizing Group of the Antiphospholipid Antibody Treatment Trial. Am J Obstet Gynecol 1997;176(5):1099–100.

[11] Pattison NS, Chamley LW, Birdsall M, et al. Does aspirin have a role in improving preg-nancy outcome for women with the antiphospholipid syndrome? A randomized controlled trial. Am J Obstet Gynecol 2000;183(4):1008–12.

[12] Kutteh WH. Antiphospholipid antibody-associated recurrent pregnancy loss: treatment with heparin and low-dose aspirin is superior to low-dose aspirin alone. Am J Obstet Gyne-col 1996;174:1584–9.

[13] Rai R, Cohen H, Dave M, et al. Randomised controlled trial of aspirin and aspirin plus hep-arin in pregnant women with recurrent miscarriage associated with phospholipid antibodies (or antiphospholipid antibodies). BMJ 1997;314(7076):253–7.

[14] Farquharson RG, Quenby S, Greaves M. Antiphospholipid syndrome in pregnancy: a ran-domized, controlled trial of treatment. Obstet Gynecol 2002;100(3):408–13.

[15] Cowchock FS, Reece EA, Balaban D, et al. Repeated fetal losses associated with antiphos-pholipid antibodies: a collaborative randomized trial comparing prednisone with low-dose heparin treatment. Am J Obstet Gynecol 1992;166:1318–23.

[16] Dahlman TC. Osteoporotic fractures and the recurrence of thromboembolism during preg-nancy and the puerperium in 184 women undergoing thromboprophylaxis with heparin. Am J Obstet Gynecol 1993;168(4):1265–70.

[17] de Swiet M, Ward PD, Fidler J, et al. Prolonged heparin therapy in pregnancy causes bone demineralization. Br J Obstet Gynaecol 1983;90(12):1129–34.

[18] Nelson-Piercy C. Low molecular weight heparin for prophylaxis of thromboembolic disease during pregnancy. In: Gamer P, Lee R, editors. Current obstetric medicine. St. Louis (MO): Mosby; 1995. p. 147–58.

[19] Auger WR, Permpikul P, Moser KM. Lupus anticoagulant, heparin use, and thrombocyto-penia in patients with chronic thromboembolic pulmonary hypertension: a preliminary report. Am J Med 1995;99:392–6.

[20] Gruel Y, Rupin A, Watier H, et al. Anticardiolipin antibodies in heparin-associated throm-bocytopenia. Thromb Res 1992;67:601–6.

[21] Langford K, Nelson-Piercy C. Antiphospholipid syndrome in pregnancy. Contemp Rev Obstet Gynecol 1999;11:93–8.

[22] Ensom MH, Stephenson MD. Pharmacokinetics of low molecular weight heparin and unfractionated heparin in pregnancy. J Soc Gynecol Investig 2004;11(6):377–83.

[23] Stephenson MD, Ballem PJ, Tsang P, et al. Treatment of antiphospholipid antibody syndrome (APS) in pregnancy: a randomized pilot trial comparing low molecular weight heparin to unfractionated heparin. J Obstet Gynaecol Can 2004;26(8):729–34.

[24] Noble LS, Kutteh WH, Lashey N, et al. Antiphospholipid antibodies associated with recurrent pregnancy loss: prospective, multicenter, controlled pilot study comparing treatment with low-molecular-weight heparin versus unfractionated heparin. Fertil Steril 2005;83(3):684–90.

[25] Pauzner R, Dulitzki M, Langevitz P, et al. Low molecular weight heparin and warfarin in the treatment of patients with antiphospholipid syndrome during pregnancy. Thromb Haemost 2001;86(6):1379–84.

[26] Pierangeli SS, Espinola R, Liu X, et al. Identification of an Fc gamma receptor-independent mechanism by which intravenous immunoglobulin ameliorates antiphospholipid antibody-induced thrombogenic phenotype. Arthritis Rheum 2001;44(4):876–83.

[27] Branch DW, Peaceman AM, Druzin M, et al. A multicenter, placebo-controlled pilot study of intravenous immune globulin treatment of antiphospholipid syndrome during pregnancy. The Pregnancy Loss Study Group. Am J Obstet Gynecol 2000;182(1 Pt 1):122–7.

[28] Jeremic K, Pervulov M, Gojnic M, et al. Comparison of two therapeutic protocols in patients with antiphospholipid antibodies and recurrent miscarriages. Vojnosanit Pregl 2005;62(6):435–9.

[29] Lubbe WF, Butler WS, Palmer SJ, et al. Fetal survival after prednisone suppression of maternal lupus anticoagulant. Lancet 1983;1:1361–3.

[30] Silver RK, MacGregor SN, Sholl JS, et al. Comparative trial of prednisone plus aspirin versus aspirin alone in the treatment of anticardiolipin antibody-positive obstetric patients. Am J Obstet Gynecol 1993;169(6):1411–7.

[31] Laskin CA, Bombardier C, Hannah ME, et al. Prednisone and aspirin in women with autoantibodies and unexplained recurrent fetal loss. N Engl J Med 1997;337:148–53.

[32] Rosove MH, Brewer PMC. Antiphospholipid thrombosis: clinical course after the first thrombotic event in 70 patients. Ann Intern Med 1992;117:303–8.

[33] Derksen RHWM, de Groot PG, Kater L, Nieuwenhuis HK. Patients with antiphospholipid antibodies and venous thrombosis should receive long term anticoagulant treatment. Ann Rheum Dis 1993;52:689–92.

[34] Schulman S, Svenungsson E, Granqvist S, and The Duration of Anticoagulation Study Group. Anticardiolipin antibodies predict early recurrence of thromboembolism and death among patinets with venous thromboembolism following anticoagulant therapy. Am J Med 1998;104:332–8.

[35] Crowther MA, Ginsberg JS, Julian J, et al. A comparison of two intensities of warfarin for the prevention of recurrent thrombosis in patients with the antiphospholipid antibody syndrome. N Engl J Med 2003;349(12):1133–8.

[36] Finazzi G, Marchioli R, Brancaccio V, et al. A randomized clinical trial of high-intensity warfarin vs. conventional antithrombotic therapy for the prevention of recurrent thrombosis in patients with the antiphospholipid syndrome (WAPS). J Thromb Haemost 2005;3(5):848–53.

[37] Kalunian KC, Peter JB, Middlekauff HR, et al. Clinical significance of a single test for anticardiolipin antibodies in patients with systemic lupus erythematosus. Am J Med 1988;85:602–8.

[38] Parke AL. Antimalarial drugs, systemic lupus erythematosus and pregnancy. J Rheumatol 1988;15:607–10.

[39] Parke A, West B. Hydroxychloroquine in pregnant patients with systemic lupus erythematosus. J Rheumatol 1996;23:1715–8.

[40] Levy RA, Vilela VS, Cataldo MJ, et al. Hydroxychloroquine (HCQ) in lupus pregnancy: double-blind and placebo-controlled study. Lupus 2001;10:401–4.

[41] Espinola RG, Pierangeli SS, Gharavi AE, et al. Hydroxychloroquine reverses platelet activation induced by human IgG antiphospholipid antibodies. Thromb Haemost 2002;87(3): 518–22.

[42] Edwards MH, Pierangeli S, Liu X, et al. Hydroxychloroquine reverses thrombogenic properties of antiphospholipid antibodies in mice. Circulation 1997;96(12):4380–4.

[43] Erkan D, Sammaritano L, Levy R, et al. APLASA Study 2004 update: primary thrombosis prevention in asymptomatic antiphospholipid antibody (APL) positive patients with low-dose aspirin (ASA). Arthritis Rheum 2004;50(Suppl. 9):S640.

[44] Kutteh WH, Ermel LD. A clinical trial for the treatment of antiphospholipid antibody-associated recurrent pregnancy loss with lower dose heparin and aspirin. Am J Reprod Immunol 1996;35(4):402–7.

[45] Triolo G, Ferrante A, Ciccia F, et al. Randomized study of subcutaneous low molecular weight heparin plus aspirin versus intravenous immunoglobulin in the treatment of recurrent fetal loss associated with antiphospholipid antibodies. Arthritis Rheum 2003;48(3):728–31.

[46] Malinowski A, Dynski MA, Maciolek-Blewniewska G, et al. Treatment outcome in women suffering from recurrent miscarriages and antiphospholipid syndrome. Ginekol Pol 2003; 74(10):1213–22.

**ELSEVIER
SAUNDERS**

Rheum Dis Clin N Am
32 (2006) 609–615

**RHEUMATIC
DISEASE CLINICS
OF NORTH AMERICA**

Index

Note: Page numbers of article titles are in **boldface** type.